A Hero's Journey
in Parenting

A Hero's Journey
in Parenting

*Parenting the Child You Didn't
Expect While You Were Expecting*

Margaret Webb

MWLC PUBLISHING

For more information, email margaretwebblifecoach@gmail.com

"Parenting the Child You Didn't Expect While You Were Expecting" is a registered trademark of Margaret Webb Life Coaching.

Author photo: Ellen Yale
Cover photo: Suzie Bailey
Back cover photo: June Bayha

ISBN 978-1-7375421-0-0 (Paperback)
ISBN 978-1-7375421-1-7 (Ebook)

MWLC PUBLISHING

Thank you AW! You have and will always be my greatest teacher. I've learned things about myself and about who I want to be because of who you are. You model so many wonderful things for me on a daily basis and inspire me to embrace the world as you do...following your passions and bringing joy to those you encounter. I love you more. ABS...always be safe.

CONTENTS

Part Seven: A Hero's Journey in Parenting Conclusion - 393

Foreword

Whether or not you were pushed reluctantly or pulled voluntarily to this point, you are here now and about to read this book. So...congratulations.

Although our accounts differ somewhat, I vividly remember when Margaret "crossed the threshold" and began her hero's journey in parenting our son. We had known about AW being autistic for several years and from a psychological standpoint, I thought we had done everything we needed to do and that the task at hand was now to support our son's development within the capabilities of his developmental differences. As we sat in a restaurant one evening together and I saw the depth of emotion in Margaret, I realized that I was wrong. In order to help AW, we also had to help ourselves.

As the pre-flight video tells you before you take off in an airplane - you have to put your own oxygen mask on first.

I can tell you first hand how deep Margaret went to find these tools she is sharing with you. From my standpoint, it was an intense journey, requiring both great strength and vulnerability. There were times where I wasn't sure where she was going or what she was going to do, but she made it back and the tools she discovered along the way are her gift to you. She would be the first to tell you that she did not invent these tools - they are timeless concepts re-forged by her particular experience in parenting. I think they could help anybody, but I know they can help parents who are struggling.

Having been there, I am excited for you. It will be difficult at times, but Margaret is a kind and loving guide. As she would also be the first to tell you, she's also funny too.

- K. Michael Webb, MD

Author's Note

Before you start reading, I feel like it is crucial to point out that my Hero's Journey in Parenting began in 2004 when autism was just starting to be discussed in the media and things were very different from what they are today.

The thoughts and feelings that I share here about autism during that time period were a direct result of the limited and "fixing" focused information available to me at the time as well as the drastic therapeutic options shared by the professionals who were part of the diagnostic process. As a mom, this was all scary and hard to hear.

In writing this book I wanted to share my honest perspective while also sharing the things that changed everything about my thoughts and feelings concerning autism and parenting a child who is on their own developmental timeline, without needing my son to be anyone other than his wonderfully awesome self.

It should also be said that ALL parents experience their own Hero's Journey in Parenting in different forms. Any parent can apply what is shared in this book when they have crossed new thresholds and feel like things are harder or not going as expected.

- Margaret

PART ONE

The Hero's Journey in Parenting

"Across the millennia of human endeavor, an archetypal narrative has emerged that describes a certain kind of transformative experience. This experience begins with an individual being confronted with a seemingly impossible challenge, typically referred to as a "call to adventure." The call to adventure is so incredibly daunting, so full of frightful unknowns, with an outcome that is so utterly in doubt, that the individual tends to resist the challenge. But eventually, the call becomes impossible to ignore and they take individual steps reluctantly into that unknown to confront the "dragon"-- the central crisis that has been thrust upon them. Scholars of this archetypal narrative have identified other stages of

the narrative, but suffice to say that, in the end, after numerous trials and tribulations, the individual meets and eventually achieves a sort of mastery over the challenge and, in the process, is transformed in a very powerful and meaningful way."

- William Webb, PhD

This narrative is known as *The Hero's Journey*, and my Hero's Journey in Parenting began like this...

Chapter One

My Hero's Journey in Parenting
The Beginning

It was 2004. I was in my early 30's and an elementary school teacher. My husband was a neurosurgical resident. We had waited to start our family and were super confident that we would have this parenting thing in the bag.

The Universe had other ideas for us and by the time our son was 15 months old, things were not going as expected. He wasn't doing what his chronological peers were doing and it was starting to spark questions from others about the possibility of autism which brought up a lot of fear, anger and confusion for me. It was during that time that we embarked on a very different parenting journey than the one we had expected while we were expecting.

I was feeling overwhelmed one day and desperately needed time to myself. I had some time between school, grocery shopping and picking our son up from daycare so I walked into Barnes and Noble and there it was again! "AUTISM" in bold print, on the cover of a magazine. I wanted to rip it from the rack, throw it on the floor, jump on it, scream and smash its existence out of my life.

Enough was enough! I was being viciously attacked by this word everywhere I went. Daycare providers brought me books about parents who did intensive treatments to cure their children. Doctors asked annoying questions like, "Does he ever make babbling sounds?" An acquaintance said, "He doesn't respond to his name. Have you considered he might be autistic?" My thoughts consisted of, "No." "Shut up." "I hate you!"

Nobody seemed to understand that he was a smart, late-talking boy like Einstein. Sure, he was not saying any consonants, did not respond to his name or wave "bye-bye" but I rationalized this by thinking that he was just intelligent and did not see the purpose. I wanted everyone to leave me and my sweet boy alone so that I could be happy again. I didn't want any part in the scary treatments or intensive therapies that were involved with an autism diagnosis.

With every comment or question made about him, I pushed down my worry, fear and anger. I ignored it all, wanting to believe that everyone was wrong. I pretended everything was fine.

I'm fine.

He's fine.

We're fine.

I pretended even though there was a quiet voice that said, "They might be right." I hated that voice. (Turns out that voice was the call to adventure and luckily it was a call for an empowering adventure that I needed badly but could never have imagined.)

Some hero's journeys are chosen and some are given to you without being asked. Either way, they forever change the course of your life. When my call to adventure arrived in the form of my autistic son, it hit me hard, like a punch in the gut. Rather than listening and answering, I wanted to pretend I had never heard it and despite it being right in my face each and every day, I ignored the call for years by keeping myself busy trying to get him to catch up with his chronological peers.

Why? In addition to thinking that it was what I should be doing, I wanted a life in alignment with what I had expected. I had followed all of the rules, I was a rule following, people pleaser after all! I wanted things to be easier...regular...normal because then I wouldn't feel like such a failure as a mother.

I loved my son more than anything. I did all I could to support him but it wasn't until I hit rock bottom, exhausted and drained of the person I used to be, that I snapped awake to some powerful discoveries of what he was here to teach me. He may need support but he was not somebody who needed to be fixed. It was not his responsibility to do or be any particular way in order to make me feel successful as a parent.

> These things I would soon discover had nothing to do with my son being autistic (or any other diagnosis or label that

> had been given to him) and everything to do with me remembering how to be curious, learning where to put my time and energy, finding and building a team and community that was supportive and non-judgmental, and empowering myself to make choices that were best for us.

I wasn't quite able to acknowledge and integrate all of those things at that point in time. In fact, I was so in my head about everything that none of that even occurred to me...that is until it got to a point where I couldn't deny that all of the energy I was spending to get him "caught up" was doing more harm than good. The reality was that he was not on a typical developmental timeline and while I was not totally ready, I swallowed my fear and took him for tests that confirmed that everyone was right. My child was autistic. I could not breathe...or think.

The moment these words, especially autism, along with ADHD, severe anxiety, sensory processing disorder and apraxia of speech, were spoken, life changed and my son went from just being my sweet child, to someone who had goals to meet and checklists to complete under the guise that this would allow him to be happy. I had crossed the threshold.

Chapter Two

Threshold Crossing

Central to the hero's journey is a threshold that creates a division between the known and the unknown, the before and the after. The call to a wild, unknown adventure is presented and there are two choices - ignore the call or answer it. It can be ignored repeatedly, denying it forever if you wish. Regardless of your choice, like it or not, there is no going back. The threshold has been crossed.

After receiving my son's diagnosis, it felt like there was no time to process. There was a sense of urgency coming from all of the specialists saying he needed a lot of help to catch up with his chronological peers so I dove into "Warrior Mom" mode. I gathered information. I researched. My research revealed more questions than answers. Any "answers" or recommendations devastated me as this was 2004 so things were very different from how they are now and none of them felt good to me.

As a Warrior Mom, I handled all the un-fun, challenging stuff so that my husband could be the fun dad he had always been. I did this because I didn't want their relationship to change and felt like I could, or rather should, carry this burden.

Honestly, my first thought was that it was because his job was demanding and when he got home, he was tired and didn't need to be bothered. However, I was working full time as a teacher, teaching all of the subject areas at different ability levels and loved my students like they were my own. This was also demanding and tiring, yet I didn't allow myself to acknowledge that at the time.

I did this all without letting anyone know how excruciatingly painful it was. This only led me to feel a tremendous amount of pressure while also tucking away any emotions I was feeling about this all. I didn't know anyone who had an autistic child so I had nobody else to talk to about this.

Sitting and playing with him felt uncomfortable because I would look at my son and feel sadness and frustration for all he was unable to do. Upon seeing this I would shift into teacher/therapist mode because I felt like I needed to fix it all asap. This turned playtime into a time I dreaded. I felt like a horrible mom for feeling these things and the vicious guilt cycle began.

All I wanted to do was to crawl back into bed and go to sleep so I didn't have those unhelpful thoughts constantly running through my mind. Instead, I took him to therapies, or therapists came to our home, while emotionally I hit rock bottom. I had nothing left to give and the excitement and expectations I had for parenting were gone.

Ultimately, I became an empty shell of a person, defined almost completely by my son's diagnosis. I had no idea who I was and just went through the motions in my tightly controlled life. I had become everything that I was trying to help my son overcome – controlling, perseverative, anxious, obsessive and isolated.

Chapter Three

Reconnecting with Myself

My son was three years old when I walked into a store and once again, a magazine caught my eye. This time instead of it being a dagger in my heart, it was a lifeline.

This magazine issue was dedicated to reconnecting people with their true, essential selves. Those words resonated in ways I didn't understand at the time but what I did know was that I needed that magazine more than anything else in my cart. I got home and devoured it like cheesecake. Here was another parenting unexpected - realizing the importance of reconnecting with myself in order to be the best parent I could be for my son. The journey back to my true, essential self began that very day.

The word "autism" comes from the Greek word "autos," and means "into one's self." I had disconnected from myself as a form of self protection from all that I made autism mean. Ironically, going into, reconnecting with and healing my essential self (the person I've always been but lost along the way) was the key to becoming the person I wanted and was meant to be. But more importantly, I could and would become the mother my son deserved.

I was especially drawn to an article about reconnecting with joy. Despite having been a happy and fun person, I hadn't truly felt joy in years as there was a part of me that wouldn't allow it.

My thinking mind told me this was selfish, but my gut told me this was exactly what I needed. It felt incredibly uncomfortable to not listen to those thoughts but I knew deep down that it was time to trust my gut. I'm glad I did because I learned so many things to help me as a parent and person.

The first thing I learned to do was press pause and do nothing. It might seem to be an odd first step, but that stillness allowed me to hear the quiet voice of my essential self once again. As I paused and did nothing, feelings and thoughts began to surface.

I learned that I had to allow myself to feel the emotions I had been repressing - anger, grief, sadness, jealousy, etc. Rather than push down those emotions as I had been doing for years, I set aside time to feel them in a way that felt safe – alone, writing letters to myself, to my son, to nobody in particular, that would be burned. I gave myself permission to express whatever came up, without judgment.

As I wrote, I sobbed for all of the times people looked at or said things about my child. My inner bitch expressed anger at not getting to choose this journey. I comforted that part of myself that needed a hug because there were a lot of times when parenting felt really hard!

I grieved for the parenting experience I had expected and expressed remorse for all of the expectations that I had placed on my son.

I wrote until I felt complete and instead of feeling stuck, which I had feared, I felt relief, clarity and acceptance. I felt hope and was able to view my child from a totally new perspective that was so much more kind and loving. I was able to "look" at my thoughts and question them which was really empowering!

What was I making autism mean? For myself? For my son?

Was any of it true?

No!

My life wasn't over. Different? Yes. Over? Nope.

My son was happy. I was not.

The miserable person I had become was not the person I wanted to be. My response to having an autistic child was to create a life of martyrdom. I did this, not autism and most definitely not my son.

This awareness was humbling yet empowering because if I could create this, I could also undo it and create something different.

I could choose my thoughts, my reactions and what I allowed into my life.

I could ask, "Is this supporting me or keeping me stuck?"

I began to add more of what felt good – people, experiences, surroundings – and subtracted what did not - mainly people who judged and support services that didn't feel good.

The power of choice expanded to all areas of my life. My son was (and still is) autistic but I was no longer controlled by my thoughts or expectations about it. I no longer attributed his unique behaviors or developmental challenges to inadequate parenting skills which made judgmental comments and looks from others far more tolerable.

The more clear and intentional I became, the more my relationship with myself and my son blossomed. I gave myself permission, time and space to care for myself and I have learned that one has to care for themselves first in order to best care for others. Not quite what society teaches AND it was only when I did this that I was truly able to see the world from his perspective and we were able to connect without my fears infiltrating our relationship.

There was tremendous freedom in knowing I could help him but that he didn't need to be fixed. Anger and frustration were replaced with deep breaths and practical strategies that work for us in our daily lives - like writing things down, using timers and daily schedules that he fills out so he knows what he is doing throughout the day - and this feels so much better.

Autism led me on this journey to go into myself, to heal, care for and notice what I need in order to be the best person and mother I can be. I crossed the threshold into this hero's journey in parenting feeling like a victim and emerged as a leader.

Chapter Four

Acceptance of the Journey

My strong hunch is that you are here because you are ready to try a different approach because nothing else is working and by now, you know that there is no going back. You are on a hero's journey in parenting.

You can choose to stay stuck, wanting what will never be and exhaust yourself trying to find the one thing that will "fix" or "cure" your child. Or, you can choose to take one step at a time into the unknown, trusting that all will be okay, that there are tools and teachers that can help you learn not only how to survive, but thrive, and feel more confident and content with the life and the child that is yours.

Despite all the noise of unhelpful and untrue thoughts that I had been accumulating, I believed deep down in my heart that my child did not need to be "fixed" or "cured" and so I chose to take step after step into the unknown. I had no idea what I was doing, but it couldn't have been any worse than what I was feeling - frustrated, incompetent and exhausted.

With each step that I took, teachers began presenting themselves with simple yet incredibly powerful tools. These tools not only helped me to reconnect with myself, they helped me to connect with my son. They helped me to not get tangled up in his big energy and emotions. They helped me discover that my son is my best teacher of all and that despite my initial feelings of inadequacy, I am actually the perfect parent for him.

> I call him our "bouillon cube child" because he inherited the most intense qualities my husband and I have as though they were boiled down to their most intense level. Intense focus. My husband! Intense anxiety. Me! Executive Functioning Challenges. Me! Persistence. My husband! (He also inherited a lot of wonderful qualities of each of us that were unfortunately overlooked back then.) Realizing this helps me to think about what we do when we are experiencing those things and support our son in utilizing the tools and strategies that we've tried rather than force him to do things in ways that would never work for either of us.

Most parents in these situations spend all of their energy in "Warrior" mode (as I did at the beginning) supporting the child, which is strongly encouraged by society and professionals. I personally found that it was crucial for me to do some things differently by taking care of myself in some unexpected ways in order to best support my son.

In addition to allowing myself to feel the emotions I had been repressing, I also became aware of all the thoughts and stories that I was believing about my son, autism and my life that were causing me pain and suffering...99% of which weren't even true! I had to realize that I was not in control of my child, his developmental timeline or simply how his brain works.

I had to reconnect with joy without putting it on hold until x, y or z happened. I will say this over and over again - I am the role model for my child of what it means to be an adult and don't most parents want their children to be happy?

The parents and caregivers that have been in my "Parenting the Child You Didn't Expect While You Were Expecting" courses as well as those I have coached 1:1 over the past 14 years come to me because their parenting journey has some sort of "unexpected," such as autism, anxiety, ADD (Attention Deficit Disorder), ADHD (Attention Deficit Hyperactivity Disorder), Dyslexia, Giftedness, SPD (Sensory Processing Disorder), PDA (Pathological Demand Avoidance or a name I prefer - Pervasive Desire for Autonomy), any neurodiversity or societal difference, which has them feeling like they are playing a never ending game of "Whack-a-Mole."

They feel judged by family, friends, teachers, therapists and even strangers for how they parent and the decisions they make. They also might feel guilty for wanting things to be different and have tried everything else but nothing else brings them what they actually want, which is to feel confident, empowered and content in the life that is their reality.

Since you are reading this, I can only assume that you love the person who led you here tremendously AND resonate with those feelings. It is my intention to leave you feeling empowered with greater clarity in order to make choices that are best for you and your family, knowing how to handle those who question and judge as well as setting boundaries when necessary.

It is my mission and passion to help you while on this parenting journey because life is too short to feel isolated, judged, uncertain and exhausted! You are NOT alone and I would be honored to be your guide and share what I have learned from the best teacher I have...my son. Throughout this all, I learned crucial lessons that I needed in order to become a more empowered person who was/is connected with what really matters in life.

The Continual Cycle of the Hero's Journey in Parenting

I hope that you will find what l share helpful in your own hero's journey in parenting. I feel like it is important to share where I began my own journey because the purpose of this book is not only to offer what has helped me most to become the parent I wanted to be for my son, but to let others know that they are not alone in what they are feeling or have felt.

The things that I share are based on my personal and professional experience as a parent, parenting coach, educator and master certified life coach with the intention of helping you to experience more ease, peace and joy in parenting.

> These are all things that made a big difference for me and my relationship with my child and I also know that everyone and every situation is unique, so take what resonates and disregard what does not.

I find that as my child gets older, new and different thresholds are continuously being crossed so I am always revisiting the tools, questions and strategies that have helped me before in order to apply them in new ways with the child I have at the time.

I want you to have access to these things whenever you need them. You can revisit them with new eyes, new perspectives and they can help you to get clarity around what is actually going on. From there, you can use your energy in effective and efficient ways in order to help yourself and your family.

Chapter Five

Archetypes in a Hero's Journey

I have debated where to place this section on Archetypes and feel like it is best to introduce them straight away since they are referenced throughout this book.

> I am NOT an expert on archetypes by any means and if this is a passion of yours, there are plenty of books written by experts. The way I present them here is simply me sharing how I learned them while wandering on this journey. I have been implementing them in my own way for the past 14 years and they have made a significant difference in my parenting.

Archetypes play a huge role in any hero's journey and while they usually show up as different characters in books and movies, they are actually energies that we have within us all of the time. The four that help me the most as a parent are the Child (East), the Warrior (South), the Teacher/Community

Builder (West) and the Monarch/Elder (North). They go hand in hand with the energy of directions on a compass, which is why I've placed directions next to their names. I'll share more about that later on as it is a super fun concept that is incredibly empowering as a parent.

Playing with archetypal energy is like stepping into a character or a role and when I was introduced to them during my nature-based coach training, I would consciously ask myself what my intention was for a given situation and how each of the archetypes could help me. Each archetype brings their own gifts and strengths and can help you to see perspectives and solutions you hadn't considered. They can help you to use energy that is more helpful and supportive to a challenging situation.

Archetypes also have what are called "shadows" and this is when there is too much or too little of that archetype's energy. What has been helpful for me has been to consider each archetype having a dial, much like those found on an old stereo system to control levels of different aspects of the music played, and since they are dials, they can be adjusted up or down. Sometimes the energy of one archetype needs to be increased or decreased in order to meet the necessary energy of the intention or the situation.

There are lots of times when an archetype goes into shadow mode and when that happens, things begin to feel out of balance. Playing with this helped me to see where I had learned, created or perpetuated unhealthy tendencies and unhelpful patterns in parenting. Good to know! Realizing this helped me recognize what was actually going on and from there, I could tap into the archetypal energies to help me parent my child with greater balance, ease and joy.

Let's dive in so that you can begin playing with this as well!

The Four Archetypes and their Shadow Descriptions:

The Child

The Child archetype is all about play, curiosity, learning and pursuing passions. It is helpful as it reminds you to be curious and to consider what your intention is for whatever you are doing. This archetype is not bound by doing what is known but is open to lots of possibilities and inspiration.

Too much of the Child archetype involves being too unrealistic about what is actually possible in a situation, not wanting to have or take any responsibility, jumping from one thing to another without following through and/or handing everything over to the "experts" without concern.

Too little of the Child archetype involves not being curious at all, having no joy or passion in one's life and/or feeling like one is wearing horse blinders with limited perspective.

The Warrior

The Warrior archetype is helpful in order to get stuff done and to set and protect boundaries. This archetype is focused on details, actions, supporting and defending.

Too much of the Warrior archetype is being too forceful and defensive, having intense focus when it is not needed, always being busy doing/defending/protecting regardless of exhaustion and is controlling.

Too little of the Warrior archetype looks like having no boundaries and allowing others to walk all over you, saying yes when you want to say no and not having clarity about the big picture which results in being wishy-washy in decision making.

The Teacher/Community Builder

I've taken some creative liberties here and call this one the Teacher/Community Builder because it seems to resonate best for the parents I coach. This archetype is focused on bringing people together to share, inform, as well as to celebrate and care for one another.

Too much of the Teacher/Community Builder archetype involves spending too much time trying to educate everyone whether they want to listen or not. Too much of this archetype may also look like needing others to agree with or do similar things you've decided to try in order to validate your choices.

Too little of the Teacher/Community Builder archetype looks like isolating and feeling like you have to do everything yourself. There is often little trust that others will understand and not judge as well as a feeling like you are never doing anything right and that everyone else knows better.

The Monarch/Elder

The Monarch/Elder archetype is helpful in order to see the big picture of what is best. This archetype is able to take a step back, removing themselves from the drama of the past, present or future concerns in order to make decisions about what can be done or tried. The Monarch/Elder utilizes the experience and knowledge that you have and also can employ the other archetypes to help you with your greater purpose.

Too much of the Monarch/Elder archetype looks like controlling and micromanaging everything as well as not being open to what others have to say unless they are deemed to be "experts."

Too little of the Monarch/Elder archetype involves not making any decisions, being wishy-washy about what to do, not trusting yourself to use the experience and knowledge that you have, but rather handing over your power and decision making to others, even non-experts.

Having these archetypes while you wander the unknown can be good to know and so helpful in noticing times when you are in shadow (too much or too little) and from that awareness, you can decide what you need to do to get back into a healthy balance of that archetype's energy in order to feel better about how you are showing up as a parent.

As I stated before, this was just a brief introduction to the archetypes and we will be getting to know them and how they support us or hold us back as parents as we proceed.

Margaret-ism
"Good to know!"

My husband and I came up with this phrase as a code for us when we notice that one of us (or both of us) is in a pattern that is not productive or helpful. One of us will say, "GTN!" and that allows that person to pivot and get back on track without defensiveness or embarrassment because there is no further discussion. For us, GTN or "Good to know" means, "I know. I'm going to try something different and I don't want to talk about it."

Note - We know that "know" is spelled with a "k" but we liked the way that GTN sounded better than GTK, so it stuck.

You will see me write "Good to know!" many times throughout this book because it comes in extremely handy in parenting both for myself and for my son. I say it when I notice an unhelpful pattern such as trying to control, and regardless of whether or not this is happening in my mind or in my actions, rather than continuing with something that isn't going to work or beating myself up, I say, "Good to know!"

This simple awareness changes everything because from there I can press pause, take a deep breath and do something different. I can use one of the tools I share to help me shift from a mindset of trying to control (Warrior in shadow) to one that is more curious (Child). I can ask that reframing question in another way like, "What can I do to influence this situation in order to support me so that I can better support my child?" This always feels better, which is good to know!

Part One Conclusion: Summary, Key Concepts and Power Questions

Summary:

The Hero's Journey in Parenting involves crossing the threshold into the unknown and has the potential to teach you things about yourself that you may never have known. Autism led me on this journey to go into myself, to heal, care for and notice what I need in order to be the best person and mother I can be. I crossed the threshold into this hero's journey in parenting feeling like a victim and emerged as a leader.

Key Concepts:

- Threshold Crossing
- Reconnecting with Oneself
- Bouillon Cube Child
- Four Main Archetypes and How They Can Help or Hinder You Along the Journey (Monarch/Elder, Child, Warrior, Teacher/Community Builder)
- Margaret-ism: Good to Know

Power Questions:

- What am I making this mean?
- Is doing x or thinking y helping me or keeping me stuck?
- What would I like to add in order to have more peace, ease and joy?
- What can I subtract in order to have more peace, ease and joy?
- What can I do to influence this situation in order to support me so that I can better support my child?

PART TWO

Why is Parenting Exhausting and What Can I Do About It?

Even if you began your journey years ago, the threshold into the unknown of parenting has been crossed. You may feel exhausted, or can remember feeling that way, when all that you've been doing isn't giving you what you thought it would. Why is that and what is causing the exhaustion?

In my experience, I have found that being in non-stop Warrior mode is a major cause. Let's explore this so you can begin to reclaim your power and energy.

Chapter Six

Non-Stop Warrior Mode

Oftentimes, the first formal diagnosis or label that your child is given or a challenge that they experience can send you into "Warrior" mode. As described earlier in the Archetypes section, the Warrior is really good at focusing on details, getting things done and defending, setting and protecting boundaries. However, there can be too much or too little Warrior energy spent in any situation, which ends up creating an imbalance.

When there is too much Warrior energy in parenting, there is intense focus on things that might be perceived as needing to be fixed and can manifest in non-stop researching. It can also look like always staying busy doing/defending/protecting regardless of the situation or the exhaustion that one experiences. Too much Warrior energy also involves attempts at controlling everything going on, which isn't possible and drains a ton of energy.

Too little Warrior energy is also not ideal because it involves handing over your power to others, having no boundaries and allowing others to walk all over you. This might look like saying yes when you actually want to say no or disconnection and lack of clarity with the big picture intention of what you want or need. This results in energy that feels wishy-washy, something others can pick up on, including your children.

I spent a lot of the early years with my son toggling between too much and too little Warrior energy. I experienced the frantic seeking and researching (the "frantic" energy being too much Warrior energy) that began immediately after he was diagnosed. I felt confused in this totally foreign space of doctors, specialists and other "experts" which led me to a tendency of handing over my power and doing whatever they said, even when in my gut, I knew it wasn't what was right for us.

I had questions for the doctors, specialists, therapists and psychologists that I wanted answered so I could wrap my head around what the future might be like for us.

- *Will my son be able to go to school?*
- *Will he be able to have a conversation with us?*
- *What will x look like when y happens?*
- *Will he have friends?*
- *Will he be independent?*

They couldn't answer any of these for me and when I reflect on them, for the most part all of these questions boil down to two central fear-based questions...

- *How do I get us back to the life I expected as a parent?*
- *Will my child be okay?*

The battle had begun, my Warrior archetype was activated and all of my energy was spent fighting this thing that had turned my world upside down. (Keep in mind that all of this happened inside of my brain despite the fact that my child was exactly the same person he was prior to any diagnosis or label.)

Does this feel or sound familiar? Going into survival mode with Warrior energy is common when things, like parenting a child who is on their own developmental timeline or one who simply marches to the beat of their own drum, start going in unexpected directions.

It makes sense to want a plan of action, to learn more about what you can do to support your child and still want to be able to perform everyday life tasks. The Warrior can be extremely useful when boundaries need to be set or things need to get done; however, living that intensely focused energy day in and day out is exhausting and not sustainable.

When I learned my son was autistic, my Warrior went into serious overdrive and I turned into a total control freak! Why? As I stated in the Author's Note, what was known about autism back then was very different from what it is now with the energy and intention primarily to "fix" or "cure" the child. None of this felt good and I was scared for what his future would/could be like.

ABA (Applied Behavioral Analysis) was the norm and pretty much the only therapy option suggested by experts. (We had an incident where a highly recommended ABA therapist forced our son to eat a piece of hot dog that he had gagged up because she didn't want him to think he won the power struggle she claimed he was in with her. She was the one in the power struggle. He had and continues to have sensory challenges with food. We didn't see her again.)

Strict and restrictive diets with endless supplements were recommended but they all either contained food he wouldn't eat or restricted him from eating the foods he would eat, not to mention that he couldn't swallow a pill.

Discussion of chelation (a process where blood is filtered to remove mercury) was prevalent among parenting groups.

Institutions were where autistic people were sent because experts didn't quite know what else to do.

Any books out there that were given to me were focused on "fixing" or "curing" the child.

In addition to the confusion and tension fueled feelings that those things brought, I craved some semblance of normalcy and calm because I knew all too well what it was like when things went awry. I would try and control all that I could from the moment he woke up until the moment his melatonin would kick in so he could finally go to sleep.

I became an obsessive worrier because it was something I could do, a way to direct the energy I was feeling, even if it didn't feel good. I prepared for the worst in order to protect myself from the intensity of his meltdowns and tantrums. The constant mental and physical energy spent trying to anticipate and control everything in our lives was draining and it turned me into a person I no longer recognized.

I eventually learned that the reality is that I cannot control anything but my thoughts and actions. You might think you can control your child or that other lucky people can control their children, but that is all just an illusion or delusion on their part.

Don't believe me? Think about it for a minute. I will bet that you can find evidence for how you planned something perfectly with controlling energy and something still went wrong.

Example:

We were in Disney World and at that point in time, my son loved ceiling fans and loved to videotape them. Unfortunately for me, Disney World has a ton of different kinds of fans and he decided that he needed to videotape them all. The first few times we had to stop what we were doing so he could do this was fine, but after that, it began to create a lot of tension for us all.

I came up with a plan where he could pick a certain number of fans from each park and since he has a great memory for things like this, he knew exactly which ones he wanted to do. He also wanted to video the fans at the bus depot in front of the Magic Kingdom, which has approximately one bazillion ceiling fans. I told him that I would do this with him if he earned it and he did.

The next morning, we set out to video the bus depot ceiling fans. I felt great, had a plan for how long he could do each one, and was excited to get this over with and get into the park to meet up with dad. About 40 minutes later, he yells out and says that we need to go back to the beginning and start over because he ran out of room on his phone. I offered my phone but he said it needed to be a continuous video.

I thought I had thought of everything. I tried to control as much as I could but still something slipped through my super-plan. Ultimately, I gave him the choice of using my phone or not filming them at all. After a brief meltdown, he chose to use my phone. Now I know to inquire about phone storage, battery level and being more specific before doing things like this.

This example, and many others like it, always remind me that I am not really in control, no matter how much I think I am. While it might feel like you are being proactive, control has a distinct tight, rigid, narrow - "blinders on" - kind of energy. Noticing this can allow you to pause and shift into a more curious "blinders off" approach in order to see if there is anything in the situation that you can influence and this feels much more expansive.

The seemingly subtle shift from control to influence means you can actually be more effective with your energy and attention. You can see options, choices, possibilities to try and with children who are not content to be placed "in the box," this approach is what is most helpful.

Believing the illusion that you should be able to control your child will eventually cause pain and frustration directed both at yourself and your child. You will beat yourself up over what you did wrong or what you could have done differently. You will increase the Warrior energy the next time to try and control even more, which usually leads to your child's Warrior ramping up to meet and beat your energy, because yes, we all have that energy within us.

The Warrior often clamps down with control and can create tension with anyone who tries to interfere with the plan/schedule/routine/etc. The Warrior means well and is just trying to keep you safe from situations that are painful and/or uncomfortable. It is an important part of who you are and it is my intention to support creating a different relationship with that part of yourself so that you can feel empowered and able to shift to more helpful and productive uses of your mental and physical energy. This is where using the other archetypes to support the warrior can make a huge impact on your life.

Balancing the Warrior Archetype with Other Archetypes

The Monarch/Elder Archetype

The Monarch/Elder archetype's superpowers involve seeing the big picture and removing themselves from the drama of past, present or future concerns in order to make informed decisions. Your Monarch/Elder archetype has the ability to tap into and utilize the experience and knowledge that you have while also knowing when to employ your other archetypes when their superpowers are best for the situation at hand. (This is SO much fun to play with, trust me!)

Noticing when your Warrior is feeling a little too controlling or intense and then checking in with your Monarch/Elder archetype can help you to utilize them both to the best of your advantage. This results in less exhaustion because there is more purposeful use, or conservation, of energy.

It can feel awkward at first, especially if you've been in non-stop Warrior mode for a while but just because something feels comfortable or normal doesn't mean it is serving the best interest of you or your family.

The Child Archetype

The Child archetype is one of my favorites primarily because I had lost connection with the energies that it holds. It's superpowers involve curiosity and viewing life experiences through a lens of play, not work. Reconnecting with this archetype gave me hope and inspiration once again as a parent.

The ability to tap into curiosity as a parent is pure gold! Utilizing questions in order to see things from different perspectives means that there is learning and growing taking place. This is quite a different experience from resorting to doing what works for others and succumbing to judgments and assumptions.

It also helps one to be open to lots of different possibilities for how things can look and be, something that is extremely relevant when parenting isn't going the way you expected. It does so by encouraging creativity in problem solving rather than resorting to what has been done in the past.

My parenting experience is nothing like I expected but by utilizing the things I will be sharing with you throughout this book and being open to approaching things in ways that are best for my son and our family, we are able to meet him where he is, shifting when necessary as he gets older. My favorite part of this all is that he is able to be exactly who he is with pride and joy.

When you model the energy of curiosity and play for your children, they get to see what it looks like to try something, have it not go as expected and learn from the feedback that is given in order to try something different the next time.

Work vs Play - An Important Shift in Perspective

Work in the sense of "I need to work on this" or "I am going to work on that" is a four letter word for me because it feels pressure-filled and is like there is a right and wrong way to do something. It is like approaching things with blinders on, not able to see other options. When that is the case there is little room for trial and error because the perceived stakes are high with a pass/fail mentality.

On the other hand, *play* allows for trial and error which provides feedback in any scenario on what works and what doesn't in order to do things differently the next time. Weaving *play* into parenting removes a lot of the heaviness that can accompany feeling like things have to be done the right way, the first time, or we are going to mess up our children.

What I find fascinating about this work vs play perspective is that we begin life being curious because it is how we are wired to learn. As we get older and enter schools that place their focus on producing good test results rather than true learning, it becomes less safe for those of us who are social, approval-seeking beings to take risks by thinking outside of the box, possibly being wrong by playing around with new ideas or different ways of approaching things. That is when the work mentality takes over and the blinders go on.

It is not a surprise to me that a lot of our children resist being placed in the metaphorical box of other people's expectations. While this resistance can be stressful to both parent and child (especially when it occurs in the school setting with its "one size fits all mentality"), I find it enlightening, and extremely helpful, to reframe this resistance as a sort of guidance our children are offering us - "this box doesn't work for me and I can't do it just to be doing it. Can we try this a different way?" Framing resistance this way engages me to do things differently, get curious and play with different ways of being and doing in order to support them in building the gifts and talents that they possess, at the pace that they are ready for.

I will now step off of my soapbox and share a basic process that will come up time and again throughout this book to help you to implement a more play-based perspective in almost anything you do.

When you create a plan for your child/family or get an idea of something to try with your child/family and then implement it with a play mentality, it creates an opportunity for learning regardless of how things go, specifically when you use three of my favorite questions...

- *What is working?*
- *What isn't working?*

- *What could be done differently the next time to help things go more smoothly?*

I learned this approach from my nature based coaching mentor Michael Trotta while trying to build a one match fire. We were at a coaching retreat, in an area that was safe for fire building, and for this activity we were asked to gather materials and assemble them in such a way that we would be able to get the structure to light with just one match. When we felt we were ready, we would receive a match, light it and see what happened.

This activity is simple yet incredibly powerful from a coaching perspective because it allows people to see patterns of how they approach something, shining a light on how these patterns show up in other areas of their life. It can illustrate a multitude of patterns, such as...

- *perfectionism*
- *levels of awareness around what is and isn't working*
- *trust or lack thereof in one's own knowledge and experience*
- *utilizing different techniques based on the current circumstances or relying solely on what has been done in the past*
- *the big picture of how one approaches a project or task*

It is a fascinating coaching tool and always has a lesson for the person building the structure.

> Awareness of patterns can actually take place anytime you are engaged in an activity or process to do something. Think of this the next time you are putting something together (like a piece of furniture or your Christmas tree), having a party or cleaning/organizing a space. Notice and reflect on your process from start to finish and then think about what you could do to make it more effective, efficient and in alignment with what you want it to feel or be like.

Because I was fully engaged in this one match fire building task and my approval seeking self wanted to get it right, to get the gold star, I attempted this exercise, which I'd never done before, with a total work mentality. I gathered up all of the Midwestern, determination-fueled energy I had and dove in head first without pausing to think through what I was actually needing in order to make this happen.

Not surprising that despite the amount of energy I put into it, there was no fire. Where else did this pattern show up in my life? Everywhere!!

When Michael presented these questions, I was able to see things from a whole different perspective.

What was working?

Not much other than the match lighting.

What wasn't working?

The sticks were too thick and the leaves too waxy which is why they weren't lighting.

What could I do differently?

I could play around with different materials in different sizes and textures to see what happened. Sure enough, after a short amount of time doing it this way, I was able to get my fire structure to light!

This experience stuck with me and I began to apply it in parenting. This concept alone has created change for us in the most positive ways. Things don't always go perfectly but modeling for my son that this is okay has helped him to be more flexible because there are always other things to try, we just need to be open and curious about what they could be.

Start checking in with yourself to see if you are approaching things from a *work* perspective or a *play* perspective and notice if it makes the same difference for you as it does for me.

Zoom Out and Zoom In

As mentioned before, when parenting became more and more unlike what I had expected, I went into full blown Warrior mode. Just like my initial one match fire attempt, I thought that if I just tried harder and focused more intensely on those things that were out of my control, things would improve. This was all well-intentioned but it kept me from truly seeing what was actually taking place right in front of my eyes.

Fortunately, I began to realize the importance of viewing situations from the Child archetype's curiosity driven perspective as though I had a "zoom out" and "zoom in" feature in my brain that I could toggle between, just like the map app on a phone. This changed my whole approach to parenting!

When things got tough, I felt like I was only able to recognize what was annoying, frustrating, different, etc. However, when I began to notice, pause and zoom out, I was able to shift and access a broader perspective which allowed me to be curious about what was actually going on.

This helped me to see what I couldn't see when I was in the thick of it...primarily what was most likely underneath or behind the surface behaviors that were causing my annoyance and frustration. It was only then that I was able to notice things such as sensory overload, emotional regulation challenges and executive functioning skills that still needed more direct support OR sometimes there were signs that he was trying to engage me in a power struggle. Good to know!

With that information, I could then zoom in and explore what I could do in that moment to influence the situation to support him and myself. This was very different from what I would have tried had I not zoomed out and seen things from a different perspective. Chances are I would have gotten frustrated and angry with him, myself and anyone else involved, followed by feelings of guilt and shame.

Curiosity around all of the parts and pieces that made up any given moment by considering what might be going on with or for him felt like such a "blinders off" experience. Things began to feel more like a puzzle to solve and I could try different things to see what was a better fit for us all at that moment. This was incredibly empowering!

The ability to zoom out and zoom in has the potential to shift the perspective, engagement and energy of even the most challenging times. The more I play with this, and I still get plenty of opportunities to do this, the easier it gets to notice patterns. This doesn't just help me, it helps us all to cycle through them faster without getting stuck in the "muck of suck."

Margaret-ism
"Muck of Suck"

The "muck of suck" is a phrase I came up with years ago when I was just beginning my coach training and doing lots of self-coaching around thoughts and patterns that were not serving me any more. I noticed that there were times when things were challenging and I was still clunky with the process of zooming out and zooming in. Everything felt hard and heavy and like I was trying to make my way through thick, goopy muck.

I was exploring why this was and what was actually going on when this phrase came to me. I was stuck in the muck of suck! I was still relying on working hard, doing things the way I was raised or employing ways that worked for some kids but not mine, and none of this was working. Since the energy I was putting out wasn't getting me anywhere, I found myself stuck in telling stories to myself, and anyone who would listen, about how tough and chaotic my life was which often led to some empathy, which felt reassuring.

This well-intentioned feedback was a "shadow pay-off" because it allowed me to have an extended pity party and to feel like a martyr. What became fascinating was that it was actually serving me in a way, not a great way mind you, but I was getting something from it just the same. It was a form of self protection and control in a way, like if I share these stories, no one can judge me or my parenting.

At the beginning of the hero's journey in parenting, soliciting empathy in this way may well be a normal, even reasonable self-protection strategy. But eventually, the "shadowy" side of this strategy reveals it to be an unhelpful crutch that prevents us from seeing our situation from different perspectives - ones that would help us all learn and grow and, occasionally, to even be able to step back and laugh at the chaos that is often our life.

Recognizing when I was in the "muck of suck" was important because it allowed me to check in to see if that's really where I wanted to be. Sometimes I did need to have a pity party for a few moments, but oftentimes I would start and after a few seconds it became clear that it wasn't actually helping me or the situation that led me there. Good to know because then I could get curious about what I could play with to influence the situation…and that felt freeing which is the opposite of feeling stuck in the muck of suck.

I could also recognize patterns or situations that would send me there and if needed, reach out to someone who could help pull me out. This is where the final of the four basic archetypes can shine.

When the Teacher/Community Builder Archetype is Not Balanced

I like to call this archetype the Teacher/Community Builder because their energy is helpful in educating and building community, something important for parents on this journey. When this archetype is balanced, it is focused on bringing people together to share information, to care for one another as well as to celebrate any and all "wins."

Being mindful and intentional about how this energy is used and who it is used with can make a difference in how you feel and the decisions you make about which relationships are worth your valuable time and energy and which are not.

> Building a team of people who can support you without judgment and/or jumping into "fix it" mode can make a world of difference. This involves relinquishing control, something that makes our Warrior very nervous, but when done with intention, can be a great source of supportive community for us and our children. We will explore this later on in greater detail.

In parenting, too much of this particular archetypal energy looks like spending time and energy trying to educate anyone and everyone about your child whether they want to listen or not. It also can look like needing everyone to agree with or do what you are doing in order to validate the choices you've made.

Wandering in the many unknowns of parenting can bring up worry, self doubt and a sense of urgency about doing the "right" thing to get your child "back on track" with their peers. When others make the same choices as you about their therapies, doctors, medicines, supplements, etc., it can feel like confirmation that you are making the 'right' choice for your child. It is important to note that what is good for one child or family isn't always what is good for another.

I can vividly remember verbally vomiting on anyone I met, sharing that my son didn't talk and that he was autistic. I now realize that I did this as a form of protection - I'll put this all out there straight away so that others can't hurt me or him with their comments and questions about why things look different.

Seeking validation from others, while totally normal, can be a shadow of Warrior energy. The tools I will share with you will help you decrease your need for others' validation and promote greater comfort with and confidence in who you know your child to be. In this way, the insensitive comments and questions that people sometimes carelessly make don't have the same intense power to sting and you can cycle through the normal feelings that can accompany those comments and questions faster.

I also spent the first few years of my parenting journey with too little of the Teacher/Community Builder energy and for me this looked like isolating myself and feeling like I had to do everything. I had little faith that others would understand

and not judge. What would people think of me, of us, if they saw how things actually were?

Sadly, I had plenty of experiences with strangers that provided evidence to support this which led to feeling like I was never doing anything right and that everyone else knew better.

Example:

There was one time in particular when I was in the grocery store needing to get one thing...dog food. The dog food was in the same aisle as the paper products and as we walked up the aisle, someone pulled off a package of paper plates and a small piece of paper came floating down like a leaf falling slowly from a tree.

Well, my son was terrified of insects, including butterflies, and thought it was an insect. He literally looked like a cartoon character climbing air while screeching in terror. I held his legs and a woman walked up and said to him, "You're too old to be acting like this." I looked at her and said, "That's not helpful."

I got his shaking body back into the cart, grabbed the dog food as quickly as I could and made a beeline to the checkout. We passed her again and she shook her head, rolling her eyes at us. I paid with tears welling up to the top of my lower eyelid and once we got to the car, I got him buckled into his seat and I bawled.

If that were to happen now, I would know that with someone like that, no words spoken in that moment could have been enough to shift whatever it was that she was feeling high and mighty about, thinking she could just plug into the situation and shame him into not having a strong reaction.

This experience, as painful as it was, taught me something crucial - I cannot waste my energy trying to get everyone I encounter to understand the challenges we face. In moments like that, my energy is best spent caring for myself and my child.

Little did I know back then that I had everything I needed to be the best parent I could be for my son. He was here to teach me how and I just had to stop worrying about everyone else and learn from him.

The Judgment Lens

Having a child who is on their own developmental timeline, has learning differences or simply marches to the beat of their own drum, can cause you to view life through a lens that magnifies their behaviors, idiosyncrasies and abilities. It can feel like living in a fishbowl with others watching and judging everything.

Judgment can become woven into even the most basic situations, like wondering what the other vacationers at Disney World were thinking as my 8-year old son laid on the ground in the United Kingdom at EPCOT Center because he didn't have the same agenda as his parents. He wanted to see lights and fans and didn't want to listen to the Beatles cover band. Judgment can create a hyper-awareness around what your child is or is not doing.

You might begin to filter everything through thoughts you create about what you think other people might think of your child or of your parenting skills. This is all mentally exhausting and often utilizes physical energy as you try to avoid judgment from others by trying to stop your child from being the way they are in the moment because people are stopping and staring.

> Human beings are wired to judge, especially when things look different. I will dive into this more later on but it has been a helpful reminder for me to practice not making it mean anything more than that when people do stop and stare at us because there were actually things my son did that looked and sounded different. I now try to tell myself, they are just being humans trying to make sense of something they aren't familiar with or don't understand.

Whenever I would try to get my son to stop a behavior I thought others would stare at, it always led to the opposite of what I wanted, an escalation of behavior, because he didn't want to be controlled AND there was always an underlying reason or cause for what he was doing. He didn't (and still doesn't) give two hoots about what other people thought of him. This was my problem and yes, I am envious of him.

I also want to acknowledge that this wasn't purely something my mind created. There were many times when those around us didn't hold their judgment back and would stare, raise their eyebrows, give dirty looks and make rude comments. None of this was helpful and left me feeling worse as a parent when what I was needing was compassion and empathy for both me and my son.

This focus on judgment is essentially handing over your power to others and making what they think more important than what you know to be true. I learned that approaching my child with judgment did not change anything and certainly didn't give me what I was wanting, which was mainly for him to stop doing whatever he was doing that was drawing unwanted attention from those around us. I wasn't aware of this until I began to notice my tension fueled thoughts and how my strong reactions created more of what I was trying to avoid in the first place.

Being in this kind of fishbowl of judgment is draining but by becoming aware of what is actually going on, of what you are making things mean about yourself, your child, your life, etc., you can take back your power, trust yourself and also not give two hoots what other people think, regardless of what they do or say. In doing so, your mental and physical energy can be used in more effective and efficient ways to support yourself and your child.

I believe that our children are here to teach us that they are all in their own individual lanes so to speak and the best way to support them is to do what is best for them... even if it looks different from what everyone else around you is doing.

Judgment is a "Hindering Force" and I will go into greater detail about later on because it is a major obstacle to finding peace, ease and joy for many on the hero's journey in parenting.

Chapter Seven

Reconnecting with What Feels Best for You

Throughout your parenting journey so far, you may have been wandering here and there, with your archetypes energies in levels of too much or too little, doing what others recommended and finding that you have lost clarity around what feels best for you, your child, your family and your life. You may have been parenting through the perspective that all of your time, energy and attention needs to be placed on your child out of fear that not doing so will cause their learning and growth to suffer.

When my journey began, I did not allow any time or attention for myself. Self care was simply not a priority. This is something that is very common with parents and can stem from what I call "internal rules."

Internal Rules

Internal rules are things taught directly or indirectly about how something or someone "should" be, what they "should" behave like or what they "should" do. This includes internal rules for yourself and other people.

I should or shouldn't do xyz even though…

But guess what? Internal rules are not set in stone. They can change. They can be broken. They can be ignored! How awesome is that?!?!

In order to be the best parent I can be for my son, I have learned how to question and oftentimes override my internal rules in order to figure out what is best for him and for our family.

> My friend Marna Wohlfeld describes this concept as though it is like replacing or updating the software that came preloaded on your computer and I love it!

While it didn't happen overnight and I had to be aware of when I was still listening to those rules. Things began to change for the better when I started asking myself two simple questions…

- *What do I want? (What is my intention?)*
- *Why do I want it? (What is my motivation?)*

I learned these from Michael Trotta as part of his inner tracking process and find that questioning one's internal rules, and basically any "should" statement, is important. Using these questions can help you get clear on what matters to you and why it matters. They can serve as powerful guideposts, most helpful when you feel like you've lost your way, you're confused or you don't know what to do next.

The internal rules that you've been carrying around for perhaps your whole life may make you feel anxious about even asking these questions. This may rock your world as much as it did mine, which is awesome! It might leave you a bit panicked because when you take a moment to think about it, you realize that you don't even know who you are anymore. If you have been disconnected from yourself, perfect!

What is perfect about this? It is perfect because this is a wonderful place to start reconnecting with your internal guidance system, beginning with those two very important questions...

- *What do I want?*
- *Why do I want it?*

> Let me be explicitly clear in that I am not talking about focusing solely on yourself and abandoning your child to figure out life on their own. Not at all! I do all I can to support my son's learning and growing AND shifting my perspective back to myself and making decisions based on what felt best for our reality helped me become a much better parent for him.

Margaret-ism
"What's Perfect About This?"

"What's perfect about this?" is one of my favorite questions, especially in challenging situations with and surrounding our children. Usually during these times our Storyteller, a character we will get to know, is busy creating and gathering up all sorts of stories and thoughts about how awful the present moment is, what other people "should" or "shouldn't" be doing or saying, and it all becomes quite believable because our Storyteller can be rather convincing.

Asking yourself this question creates a little pause and puts our incredibly creative thinking mind to work searching for how this experience could be perfect, not in the sense of faking how awesome or ideal something is, but rather playing with curiosity around what this experience could be helping you to practice, play with, or learn.

- It could be a perfect time to set boundaries.
- It could be a perfect time to say "No" or "Yes" to something.

- It could be a perfect time to get clarity around what really matters in the moment in order to focus on that.

- It could be a perfect time to allow yourself some time and space to feel emotions you might resist feeling.

- It could be a perfect time to laugh at the ridiculousness of what is happening and not take everything so seriously.

- It could be a perfect time to play with doing something different since nothing else is working.

- It could be the perfect time to ask for help despite thoughts that you "should" be able to do it all on your own.

Using this question can help you shift perspective regardless of what is happening in order to best support yourself as a parent. It can also help you model for your child how to use their Storyteller in a way that is empowering as opposed to feeling at the mercy of thoughts that create additional pain and suffering.

Setting Intentions

Intention setting is very different from having expectations, primarily because expectations usually involve the Storyteller creating a detailed and specific version of how things will occur. Expectations can be rigid, limit alternative possibilities and usually involve words like "needs to" and "has to."

Expectation example:

My child needs to/should do x because that is what children their age do.

This is a challenge because we cannot control another human being's brain development or who they are as an individual.

Intentions are more generalized wants and once set, allow the brain to automatically orient itself around that intention. It becomes a mindset that shifts our perceptions, focuses our attention, clarifies our goals, and gives purpose to our actions---all in service toward realizing that intention. Setting an intention is like aiming at a target. Without that aim, hitting our target is just wishful thinking which, come to think of it, is sort of what an expectation is.

Intention example:

I want my child to learn and grow because I want them to be happy and the best version of themselves possible.

Notice the difference?

When I began my parenting journey, my mind would go blank when I asked myself, "What is my intention?" or more simply, "What do I want?"

I struggled to answer those simple questions for myself, though I could tell you what I thought my husband, our son or even my dog wanted. What I wanted? Forget about it! Even something basic like what I wanted for dinner was incredibly tough! Why was that?

Like many parents, my Warrior was trying to keep me safe by living in a defensive mode. I existed this way mentally, physically and emotionally. While I struggled with the thoughts and stories I created around what my son's life would be like, I had lost true connection to my own life.

I was tired from wandering in the seemingly never ending unknown of parenting. My Warrior felt it would be safer and less disappointing to distance myself from having wants, needs, ideas and hopes. Eventually I did not know who I was anymore without the label of "mom," "wife," "teacher," "daughter," "sister" or "friend." A huge part of my hero's journey in parenting involved rediscovering myself so I could show up and make choices that reflected my intentions as a parent.

As I shared earlier, the Warrior within us has a strong desire for safety and control. However, Warrior energy is best utilized when there is a big picture vision (the energy of the Monarch/Elder) that stems from a clear and intentional "What?" and "Why?"

I have noticed that with people who are also on a hero's journey in parenting, there is a reflexive tendency and desire to deal with, fix or make the unexpected go away as quickly as possible. This is a totally normal reaction! It is uncomfortable to have something come into your life that changes everything, including life as you expected it to be, without your permission.

How do I know this? All I have to do is go back to that day I previously described in the pediatrician's office to remember those uncomfortable feelings and the intense desire to make them go away. I had no thoughts about anything other than to do what the doctor said to do with the intention of getting him caught up with his peers.

My Warrior was activated, ready and willing to do whatever was needed to complete this mission! Evaluations were set up. Therapists deployed. Toys purchased to help build developmental skills. The battle had begun.

This was all great and while there were things we did that definitely helped him, I would call this a "shadowy" intention. It was as much a desire to get back to what I knew or expected as soon as possible as it was to support my son.

Why? I selfishly needed some proof that I was a good mom. I also wanted to show the world he was just like his peers. This may have made me feel better in the moment, but it certainly didn't allow me to see beyond the moment to who he truly was or to understand and acknowledge that he didn't need to be fixed. Supported? Yes. Fixed? Not at all!

I now know that if I would have stopped for a moment, gotten curious about what I wanted and why I wanted it, I would have seen that it all was a deep desire for my son to be happy and accepted as he is. I would have also seen that he was already happy being exactly who he was. Unlike me, he always knew what he wanted and how to get it. I just needed to accept him. Interesting twist, huh?

If you have spent a lot of time trying to get your child to hurry up and be like everyone else their age, do not judge yourself! Remember, the Warrior in us takes over to protect our ego and calm our fears. It doesn't want us to feel hurt and it is desperately trying to deliver certainty back to us.

If we can dial back a little of that intense Warrior energy, it makes answering these questions - "What do I want?" "Why do I want it?" (with the support of our Monarch/Elder) - some of the most effective guiding principles you can have.

Intention Setting When the Path Isn't Clear

Another form of control that I became familiar with involved wanting to follow the rules, the recipe, the instructions...you name it...so that I could feel like I was getting something, anything, right. This also came from the want I mentioned earlier, the desire to be considered a "good mom."

As you well know, there are no manuals that come with our children, and if there are, yikes, I must have left mine at the hospital! What I have learned is that our children ARE the manuals. The more that you can tune into them, be curious, notice and observe, you will see that they are constantly letting us know what works and what doesn't work for them.

If this is resonating, you might want to know what you can do differently.

I have learned that the most important thing to do when you feel tension around something is to press pause for a moment.

This might feel counterintuitive because there is a desire to take action, however, pressing pause can help you to get curious around what is actually going on in the moment – thoughts, stories, frustrations or annoyances. This is all good to know so that from there, you can check in with your intention for the present moment and decide what sort of attention you can give to get back on track.

When I did this, it helped me get clear about what my intentions were for myself and my son. It helped me sort out what I wanted and why I wanted it. Did I want to be loving and accepting of who he was and what parenting was going to be like? Or did my ego want him to catch up so I could have proof that I was a good mom? Was my goal for him to be happy? Or was it for him to be different from who he was in order to be like his peers?

Reconnecting with your internal guidance system that knows what feels true for you allows you to make decisions from a more empowered perspective. While it felt uncomfortable and selfish at first, tapping into curiosity around those questions "What do I want and why do I want it?" changed my life and helped me feel more clear, focused and content as a parent.

Take a moment and ask yourself these questions. It doesn't even have to be about your intentions for your child. If you have been disconnected from your true self for a while, here are some of my favorite ways for you to play in order to get started.

What do I want...

- for the next five minutes?
- for the morning/afternoon/evening?
- for dinner?
- for this grocery store trip?
- for this family gathering?
- for this holiday/season?

Why do I want this and what will it give me that I don't have?

- It will help me to feel good.
- I will feel organized.
- I will feel prepared.
- I will be able to enjoy the experience.
- I will use my time and energy effectively.

The more you play with asking these questions in basic scenarios, the more you are repatterning your brain to have them as your go-to questions regardless of the chaos and intensity of a situation.

I frequently have conversations with my coaching clients about whether or not their child "should" be doing certain therapies, going to certain schools or getting evaluations. Every single time, I go back to intention. "What" are they wanting (Are they wanting it?) and "Why" are they wanting it?

These questions invite them to find clarity by checking in with the different archetypal energies - the big picture vision of the Monarch/Elder, curiosity of the Child, boundary setting or figuring out more specific details with the Warrior and utilizing what they know about their child via the Teacher/Community Builder to support the intention.

> I hope that you are starting to see how helpful they can be in all situations!

When a client comes to me confused about a choice that they need to make, my process goes something like...

What is your intention for signing your child up for or wanting them to do x?

Why x?

How will it support your child?

Knowing what you know about your child, do you feel like it is best for them?

Is there any additional information you can provide to those involved with x that will allow you/them to best support your child?

Asking yourself these basic questions can help you to feel clear and grounded about the choices you make for your family. This feels so much more empowering than making decisions simply based on what other people are doing or telling you that you should do.

From there, you can move on to bigger questions like...

What is my intention as a parent to the child/children I have?

- It is my intention to be a parent who...

Why do I want this?

- I want this because it will help me feel...
- I want this because I want my child/children to feel...

Your intention may be wanting more connection with your child or with other people who are on a similar journey and/or acceptance from others so that you can better support your child. Or you may want parenting to feel easier and more joyful. Maybe you want your child to be happy, to learn and grow. All of these intentions are wonderful and they can help you get clear on what you need to make decisions and move forward.

You may have answered that your intention is to do what you can to make this all go away! You may feel like doing so will give you your life back. It'll make things easier and then you can be happy once again.

You would not be alone if you answered that way. If you had asked me early on in my journey, those certainly would have been my answers! It is my hope that what I share will support you in feeling happier and more content in parenting without needing your child to be any different from who they are. Sure, there might be sources of tension that would be nice to alleviate but we will get to those and some likely root causes of them later.

Pressing pause in times that feel overwhelming or chaotic allows for an opportunity to slow down, check in with intention and move step by step so that you can focus your attention on one thing at a time. This means that you are in the present moment, things actually get noticed/addressed/finished and that feels so good! It helps us all to have other desired intentions - more ease, peace and joy in parenting and in life!

Change is Possible

Change is possible, but only when there is awareness and curiosity around what is not working anymore. Having a willingness to play with other ways of being and/or doing, plus paying attention to what works and what doesn't work, will support you in adding things that create more ease, peace and joy, while taking away things that don't... for you and your family.

As I began to observe myself from this perspective, I noticed that I was all over the place - both physically and in my mind - all of the time and I began to do something different. I would press pause or slow down whenever I became aware of myself "pinballing" or "boomeranging" (more specifics on these later on). This felt awkward and uncomfortable at first but doing so allowed me to ask questions like...

- What is my actual intention for right now?
- What actually matters?
- What is actually important?
- What is actually going to be most helpful?

> I love using the word "actually" because it helps my Storyteller to boil things down to what is necessary and not create stories about what unnecessary things should distract my energy and attention.

I could then take a few seconds to check in to see if what I was doing was supporting the answers to those questions. If it was? Awesome! If it wasn't? Awesome!

Why would it be awesome if I was doing things that weren't supporting my intention? It was awesome because noticing this meant I could choose to do something else! Change cannot happen without noticing and this awareness meant that I could immediately shift my energy and attention to do things that would actually support what mattered most in that moment. All of this helped me to be more effective and efficient, to put my energy to use supporting myself, my child, my family and my home.

This helped me and it also helped me with my son because he does best when things are direct, explicit and clear. He tends to get easily distracted by things he finds more interesting, like his phone, when asked to do things like household chores or his hygiene tasks (brushing teeth, deodorant, washing face, shaving, etc.). Understanding this changed how I approach things with him.

I've come to understand that he is a visual learner and executive functioning is something he struggles with, so he does best when things are written out. I'll print things like chore lists, packing lists and daily schedules or sometimes I text him. Because he can see it, he is more likely to be able to do it. I am a kinesthetic learner, so the process of writing things down for myself plus using a timer works and when I feel like I've begun to pinball, I can go back to my list to refocus.

Can you relate to this? Do you jump into action mode without necessarily being clear about what is wanted or needed throughout the day. If so, what if you took a few minutes to set some intentions and check in with what sort of attention needs to be given to things on your schedule/calendar/agenda/to-do list.

Slowing down, checking in with intention and moving step by step works beautifully to focus attention on one thing at a time. This means that things actually get finished and that feels so good! It helps us all to have another desired intention - more ease, peace and joy!

Now that you know why you've been feeling drained and lost, let's start exploring the tools, questions and strategies that can help you to refuel, get clarity and discover strengths, possibilities and capabilities in parenting you may never have known you possess.

Part Two Conclusion: Summary, Key Concepts and Power Questions

Summary:

Once you have crossed the threshold, any threshold in life, there is a desire to find some certainty so that you can feel like you have some semblance of normalcy and control. The Warrior LOVES a mission and sets to work straight away to find the way to provide these things. Unfortunately, control is an illusion and part of the journey is learning how to allow the other three archetypes to help create greater balance so we not only stop feeling so exhausted but also can find some clarity by getting perspective on where our time, energy and attention are best spent.

Key Concepts:

- Exhaustion Cause - Non-Stop Warrior Mode
- Shifting from Control to Influence
- Utilizing Monarch/Elder Archetype to Balance Warrior Archetype
- Work vs Play - An Important Shift in Perspective
- Zoom Out and Zoom In to Gather Information from Big Picture to Details

- Margaret-ism: Muck of Suck and Shadow Payoffs
- Noticing When Teacher/Community Builder Archetype is Not Balanced
- Judgment Lens Creates Unhelpful Filter
- Recognizing Internal Rules...In Yourself and Others
- What's Perfect About This?
- Expectations vs Intentions

Power Questions:

- Is there anything about this situation that I have influence over?
- What is working?
- What isn't working?
- What could be done differently the next time to help things go more smoothly?
- What do I want? What is my intention?
- Why do I want it? What is my motivation?
- What's perfect about this?
- What actually matters?
- What is actually important?
- What is actually going to be most helpful?

PART THREE

Reclaiming Your Power

You have been introduced to common occurrences for parents who have crossed their own thresholds into their own hero's journey in parenting. These often consist of Warrior energy spent in ways that might seem productive and normal, but are actually the opposite.

In this part, you will learn about some characters that can be helpful but when they feel too important or are driving the metaphorical bus, they become Shadow Forces.

I've named these characters *the Storyteller, the Battle Ready Bodyguard, and the Guardian of Your Heart.* You will learn all about each of them individually in greater detail and how they are trying to be helpful. I will also give you tools, questions and strategies to help you take back your power when they become a Shadow Force. This is important because when they are in control, your life is full of tension. Who needs that?!

Your Warrior will get nervous about this and that is okay. It might make you feel vulnerable and that is okay. Be kind and loving with yourself. Go slowly if that feels good. Pause when necessary. Trust that this is all just a reclaiming process to take back the power and connection you've had all along. It's been kept safe, like a treasure, until you were ready and since you are here, I can only assume that now is the perfect time.

> The thoughts, feelings and emotions that come up are for you and you alone. Resistance to allowing these to come up usually comes from fear of vulnerability and fear of what they mean. If you choose to share with others, please make sure they are safe people who can listen without judgment, commentary or encouraging you to just look at the bright side. It can really sting to share something that feels important and true with someone who minimizes or dismisses it.

Chapter Eight

Shadow Force
#1 - The Storyteller

In any hero's journey, obstacles present themselves and need to be overcome in order to move forward. One of the major obstacles you will face lies not in the fact that parenting is not what you expected while you were expecting...it is with the expectations themselves.

Let me introduce you to the Storyteller, also known as your amazingly creative thinking mind, and is the part of you that creates these expectations. This ability is what makes us different from other species and is all fine and dandy until the thoughts and stories it creates begins to impact how you experience life and those in your life. I call this a Shadow Force because a lot of the time it creates unnecessary pain and suffering, especially when those thoughts, stories and expectations involve your child and your parenting.

"The mind is a wonderful servant and a terrible master."

Robin Sharma

If you've ever practiced stillness or tried to meditate, you may already have noticed the constant stream of thoughts going through your mind. Even in the avoidance of stillness, you can be curious about the thoughts that are keeping you from doing it. This is totally normal and what stunned me when I learned this was the fact that I was believing every single thought I had without question. Every single one!

Some thoughts are kind and loving. Some are harmless commentaries or reminders about things. However, if you are anything like me, many of them are judgmental, shaming, demanding and doubt fueling. These thoughts may seem like they are helpful and productive but once you start to separate yourself from them and see them more clearly, you will realize how often they do more harm than good, which is usually the opposite of what you are wanting.

Your Storyteller most likely had many ideas about what parenting was going to be like. Whether it began when the test came back positive or when you got the word that the adoption was going through. Those thoughts and stories probably included idealized versions of parenthood based on commercials or of the perceptions you had of other people's experiences. They also probably included what your child should be able to do or what they would be like.

When reality strays from those expectations, the Storyteller gets to work and creates new thoughts and stories, which often lead to feelings of shame and judgment. Creating some space between you and your Storyteller can be helpful in order to get perspective. Noticing the stories your Storyteller is telling you allows you to begin to question the thoughts. This is important because if you don't question them, they will feel normal and important regardless of the tension they create.

Pay close attention to thoughts that include the words "should," "have to," "need to," or any other language that is limiting. Those are some of the Storyteller's favorite ways of getting your attention and are also great thoughts to question with this process.

Your Storyteller will frequently take you back to situations to relive them over and over again, thinking about what "should" have been said or done. I call this "should-ing" on yourself and others and it only serves to create tension that begins in your mind and then transfers to your body. This creates physical tension in your body, so that long after an experience is over, you are still experiencing the stress of a past experience in real time.

Before realizing this was happening, I would revisit conversations and situations and "should" on myself, my son, my husband, teachers, random people in the grocery store, or those driving on the same road as me.

I began to see how often I was placing pressure on myself and others as I imposed my internal rules on them.

I should...

He shouldn't...

They should...

Should, shouldn't, have to, needs to are all key words and phrases to alert you to when you are listening to internal rules.

As I mentioned earlier, internal rules are things taught directly or indirectly to us or by other people around us about how something or someone "should" be, what they should behave like or what they should do. This includes internal rules for yourself!

I cannot rest because I should be doing something.

As a mom, I must sacrifice everything to support my son.

I must give all of my attention to my child at all times.

Your Storyteller will also take you into the future creating detailed scenarios about what "might" happen. It creates a storyline of how something "might" play out or how we or others "might" behave.

As human beings we are so gifted at using our creative brains that it feels as though things are actually happening in real time. None of these stories take into consideration that the only things we can control are our thoughts, actions and reactions in the moment.

While it is impossible to predict the future with certainty, thinking about the future as a way of considering the range of possible outcomes to some event and how you might respond to those outcomes is not unreasonable. In fact, it can be helpful under certain circumstances.

What is not helpful, however, is to let your fear of the future's "worst possible outcome" become your brain's imagined reality. This sort of "future tripping" creates tension in the mind and body (known as anticipatory anxiety) as you pre-live the fearful situation. Your body believes what your mind is experiencing. It doesn't know the difference between imagined thoughts and actual experiences. It prepares itself either way in order to protect you in whatever you are battling, even if it's fictional.

The result, of course, is that you have potentially put yourself in the unnecessarily stressful and counterproductive position of experiencing anxiety twice---first from the anticipatory anxiety and again if the outcome does, in fact, turn out to be unfavorable. What's more, dwelling on the "worst possible outcome" may, in fact, make that outcome more likely due to the "self-fulfilling prophecy" effect (the psychological process by which our expectations about some future event causes us to act subconsciously in ways that confirm those expectations).

The emotions and feelings associated with frustration, annoyance and irritation increase when we fight against the reality of what is actually going on in the present moment by believing that things "should," "need to" or "have to" be different.

I experienced my own personal lightbulb moment around my own thoughts, when I noticed that I was extremely hard on myself. My thoughts included things like...

- *I am not doing enough.*
- *I should have done this.*
- *I should be doing that.*
- *I should be doing whatever someone else is doing.*

Should. Have to. Need to. Ugh!!

I realized I expected all sorts of super-human things from myself. There were the typical "shoulds" that accompany parenting any child, however there were also a heap of extra "shoulds" that came from parenting a child who was on his own developmental timeline.

The crazy thing, or perhaps maybe the most sane thing, about these thoughts were that they were so overwhelming to think about that when I did ponder them, I felt like crawling back into bed! Because I couldn't do that and no matter what I did or tried, I had no control over the developmental timeline that my child was on, so I did what lots of people do...I tried controlling whatever I could.

I was very rigid and controlling over our daily schedule, what we ate and where we could go.

When we left the house, I obsessively prepared what I could to avoid any meltdowns, tantrums or bathroom accidents. My bag of tricks looked quite similar to a Mary Poppins bag.

> I've often joked that you would definitely want to be sitting next to me on a plane because I'll have anything you might need - food, electronics, chargers, extra clothes, straws, cups, etc.

I tried to control as much as I could in order to combat those thoughts of not doing enough, but they were always there, waiting to pounce.

When I began to notice all of those judgmental thoughts I was having about myself, I was humbled to realize that they were coming from a place of protecting myself (Warrior energy) from what others might think.

My life felt so crazy and chaotic and unlike anything I knew of anyone else's life. I was embarrassed that if anyone found out what things were really like, they would judge me and my ability to parent my child.

The reality about this all was that nobody else was actually judging me as harshly as I was judging myself. They didn't have to judge me because I was already doing it to myself. I was thinking and saying things that were much meaner than anything anyone else would say, though I've certainly had people give me comments and looks that stung.

Wandering Into Byron Katie's Inquiry Process - The Work

Recognizing the power that your thoughts have over you and taking that power back is a key lesson that can change your life. I am personally grateful that as I wandered through my own hero's journey, Martha Beck introduced me to Byron Katie's Inquiry Process known as "The Work."

Byron Katie's "The Work" led to a powerful awareness for me around not only the thoughts I was thinking and the stories I was creating about my life as a parent to my autistic son, but the impact that those thoughts and stories had on my relationship with him and others in my everyday life. They were keeping me from being able to be fully present. The reality is that the present moment is the only moment any of us can actually do anything about anything.

"The Work" is a tool created to take power away from our Storyteller when it is operating as a Shadow Force in order to question the thoughts. It consists of four questions to ask yourself when you notice a thought that causes tension. It shines a light on what happens when you believe your thoughts and can open you up to wonderful possibilities in your life. "The Work" helps you shift into curiosity and away from simply believing your thoughts as the absolute truth.

We often have the same thoughts over and over again and there are many versions of the same thoughts. As Byron Katie says, "There are no new stressful thoughts, they're all recycled."

Let's take a look at common thoughts for parents:

- *I'm not doing enough.*
- *I'm not a good parent.*
- *If I do x, everything will fall apart.*
- *They should be able to do x.*
- *They shouldn't do x.*

When you notice a tension provoking thought, try following Byron Katie's "The Work" Inquiry Process by asking...

1. Is it true? (Yes or No only because our Storyteller LOVES to find ways to "protect" us by finding evidence and giving us ways around actually getting to what we honestly think or believe. There is NO right or wrong answer, no judgment either way!)

2. If the answer to number one was Yes, ask yourself if you can absolutely know that it is true? (Again, only Yes or No)

3. Who do I become when I believe the thought? What do I do? How do I treat myself? How do I talk to myself? How do I treat those around me? How do I speak to them? What is my tone? How do I feel in my body?

4. Who would I be without the thought? If I cannot think this thought, what would I do? How would I treat myself? How would I talk to myself? How would I treat those around me? How would I speak to them? How would I show up in the world? How would my body feel?

Example:

My son should be potty trained. (This was one I struggled with when my son was five and was not doing #2 in the toilet.)

1. Is it true? *Yes*

2. Can I know that this is absolutely true? *No*

3. What happens when I believe the thought? *I get annoyed with him. I feel like I've done something wrong. I'm irritated when I have to clean things up. I'm not very kind with my words to him when he doesn't go in the toilet. I make it mean all sorts of things about his future. I'm annoyed with people who ask about it. I'm annoyed with people who have younger kids who are potty trained. My body is tense. I watch him constantly like a predator and when I notice his stomach clenching, I pounce on him to race him to the restroom which usually stops whatever process was about to happen.*

4. Who would I be without the thought? *I would be kinder to him and to myself. I would be more patient and relaxed around it all. I wouldn't make it such a big deal. I would just take care of things without all of the tension. I wouldn't care and make it mean anything more than that he's not ready. I would remember that this is about his brain development*

and has nothing to do with my parenting or of who he is as a child.

> Please be aware that there are times when you might find yourself in what is called a "blind spot" where you cannot see how and what you would be like without the thought. This is your Storyteller and ego trying to keep you safe from other fears and thoughts but actually keeps you from experiencing even the possibility of peace without the thought. If you notice this, you can jot down the other thoughts to do "The Work" on another time but I'd encourage you to stick with the original thought.

Once you've created this awareness around a thought, play around with how the opposite, or "turnarounds" as Byron Katie calls them, might be true. This is a wonderful way to put our super creative minds to use finding evidence for how this is true in order to have less tension and more ease and joy in life!!

Turnarounds for common parenting thoughts:

- *I am doing enough.*
- *I am a good parent.*
- *If I do x, everything will not fall apart.*
- *They should not be able to do x.*
- *They should do x.*

Example:

My son should be potty trained. (Original thought)

Turnarounds:

My son should not be potty trained...

- *because his brain is not ready;*
- *because the reality is that he is not and my fighting reality causes pain and suffering;*
- *until he connects the feelings involved with what needs to happen;*
- *because it is something that cannot be forced.*

Following these turnaround statements with the words "because" and "when" can be helpful if you get stuck. The ego part of our Storyteller loves to resist letting go of thoughts and will do all that it can to try and convince you to stay safe and protected under the guise of these unhelpful thoughts. The more you can create some wiggle room around them, the easier it gets.

As you begin to do this more and more, be kind and loving with yourself, especially as you may notice yourself feeling like you "should" have always been doing this. This is "good to know" because when you don't know, you can't do anything different and now you are on the path to knowing more and more!

Once you have an awareness, you can play with noticing the thoughts and stories your Storyteller creates throughout the day. You can take a deep breath, question them and empower yourself to choose those that support you in learning and growing as a parent in order to have more peace, ease and joy in all aspects of your life.

> If you want to learn more about Byron Katie and The Work head to www.thework.com.

Chapter Nine

Shadow Force #2 - Your Battle Ready Bodyguard

When your Warrior archetype is leading you on your hero's journey, part of the Warrior can take on the role of what I like to call your *Battle Ready Bodyguard*. Your Bodyguard is charged with protecting your heart and ego at any cost. It is on high alert to any sort of danger, real or imagined.

If it feels like you are under threat - even a threat that is perceived or created by the Storyteller - it will respond accordingly by preparing you to fight or flee a battle. It can also freeze up in uncertainty or nervousness.

It is not uncommon for the Bodyguard to try and keep you safe by disconnecting you from your body. The overactivation and/or disconnection from your body is when it becomes a Shadow Force.

Your Battle Ready Bodyguard has probably been on non-stop duty since the day your child entered your life or more specifically when you crossed the threshold into your Hero's Journey in Parenting, the day you noticed that your child was on their own developmental timeline, if/when your child got a diagnosis or label or when unexpected differences that strayed from societal norms emerged. It is tough to learn about something that may cause challenges or struggles for your child; the Battle Ready Bodyguard goes into battle mode to protect you.

It also works hand in hand with your Storyteller and demonstrates the incredible power of your thinking mind to be creative, imaginative and powerful enough to impact your body with physical responses, as though you are experiencing whatever you are thinking in real time.

> What always comes up for me when I think about this concept is pickles. I'm not sure if this is just me, but whenever I think about pickles, I salivate. It's like my mouth knows that it needs to counter the vinegar and salinity of pickles and so it gets ready. All because I thought about a pickle…and yes, as I write this, I am salivating.

In the last section, you learned the importance of noticing and questioning your Storyteller's thoughts. Now you will learn to recognize when your Bodyguard has taken over, believing those thoughts, and what it feels like when it is alerting you to its presence.

You may already have begun playing with this when answering the question from Byron Katie's Inquiry Process, "The Work," when answering the question, "What happens when you believe the thought?" Your body is a great indicator of when Shadowy Forces are at play. Observing your body's reactions, which we will discuss more in the next section, is a key to decoding your Storyteller's messages and uncovering your true thoughts and feelings.

The Link Between Your Storyteller's Creations and the Way You Feel

The simple act of thinking about something creates physical sensations in your body as though you are actually experiencing it in real time – positive and negative.

Just like with the Storyteller, the Bodyguard has three different ways that it goes about protecting you.

1. You can go back to the past and relive situations or conversations, thinking about what you or others "should" have done or said.

Doing this might feel productive, like you are making it right in your head and trying to be intentional and proactive about preparing for similar situations in the future. In reality, you will spend a ton of energy spinning stories as a means of judging, shaming or beating yourself (or others) up. This process actually creates the same feelings of stress and tension that you felt in the original experience. Why would you want to relive a crappy situation?

I do use a three question process mentioned earlier...

- What worked?
- What didn't work?
- What is something I can try the next time to see if I get a different result?

...however, the intention and energy of reliving past experiences and conversations from a "should have" perspective is completely different from a desire to learn and do something differently the next time based on what came from asking those questions.

We use this process for family trips and holiday planning so that we can be intentional with what we've learned from past experiences to have greater ease, peace and joy during what are often stressful situations. It feels so much better than sitting in anguish over what we "should" have done differently, especially since we have that information at our disposal.

2. Your Storyteller can go into the future and use your imagination to pre-experience a situation or conversation that you might be nervous or worried about. Your Battle Ready Bodyguard takes action and your body will respond as though you are in that future moment regardless of where you are and how calm things may be around you in the present moment.

As mentioned before, there is a difference between being proactive and intentional in order to use what you know to help empower yourself and your child.

Your Storyteller is trying to be helpful by doing this so that you feel prepared and protected, but it is essentially creating a fictional negative experience in advance. You feel like you are already experiencing it, when in actuality, the only time you can do anything about what is going on is in the present moment. Why create unnecessary pain and suffering for yourself?

3. You can be in the present moment and notice that if you are feeling tension or tightness, your Battle Ready Bodyguard has probably jumped into action in order to protect you. This is when it is super helpful to get curious about what your Storyteller is trying to tell you about the present moment. Tension in the body typically occurs when a lot of "should-ing" is taking place.

Common examples of this are...

- *They should...*
- *They shouldn't...*
- *I should be able to...*
- *Why aren't they...?*
- *I have to...*
- *They need to...*

The list could go on and on but it really is helpful to begin recognizing those keywords - should, have to, need to - because they almost always are your Storyteller's thoughts.

Noticing When You Are In Your Head

The act of momentarily pressing pause and getting curious about what is actually going on in the present moment, can lead you to notice if you are allowing your Storyteller to be in charge, or "driving the bus," so to speak. What's perfect about this? (Here is that Margaret-ism once again!) Once you notice that you are in your head, you can take a breath and get back into your body.

My favorite way to do this is to bring my attention to my feet as they are the farthest part of my body from my head. Doing so brings me immediately into the present moment, using my Storyteller in a more effective way, to get curious *about what is actually going on* as opposed to what it was telling me to *think* was going on. Big difference!

If you are like so many, you may be realizing that your Battle Ready Bodyguard has totally disconnected from your body. If you check in and can't connect with how they are protecting you, start super small. Do not worry and do not judge!

A wonderful and simple way to do this is to check in with your senses - What am I smelling? What am I tasting? What am I hearing? What am I feeling on my body? What am I seeing?

I love this so much because it is almost impossible to be present with your senses AND be thinking other thoughts. This is a great way to assign your Storyteller a mission (something the Warrior LOVES!) to use its gifts in a different way by thinking about what is going on in your body.

Some basic things you can do are...

- Rub your hands together slowly and notice how that feels.
- Put your hands on your face and notice how that feels.
- Put your feet on a soft carpet or towel and notice how that feels.
- Notice how different fabrics and textures feel against your skin.

Begin there and start to connect with what feels good, what doesn't, what is too tight or creates irritation or what feels comfortable and pleasant to your senses.

Body Scan

In order to start rebuilding a healthier connection between your mind and body, you can periodically do a quick scan to notice what's going on. This is something I learned during my life coach training with Martha Beck and has stuck with me all of these years.

Take a deep breath. Starting with your feet, slowly bring your attention to the different parts of your body as you move up to your head. Notice if there are any parts that are feeling tense, and if so, get curious about any specific descriptions of that tension it feels. (This gives your Storyteller and Battle Ready Bodyguard something productive and helpful to do by putting language to what you are actually feeling rather than creating stories about its perceptions.)

Quite often, people feel tension in their:

- shoulders
- neck
- jaw
- chest
- hands
- stomach

Here are some common descriptions that people link to tension fueled thoughts:

- tension
- tightness
- clenching
- heat
- shallow breathing
- heaviness

If you notice anything, such as tension or tightness, ask yourself...

- *What is actually going on?*
- *Where are my thoughts?*
- *What am I trying to protect myself from or prepare myself for?*

The simple act of a quick body scan along with those basic questions can empower you with insights into how your Storyteller and Bodyguard are trying to help you (even in their misguided Shadow Force ways). You will also have a greater awareness of how this can drain your energy keeping you from actually being present and able to use your energy and attention in ways that are effective.

When I began playing with this in my life, there was one specific incident that sold me on this concept. I was alone in my car, driving to pick up my son from school, and then we were off to his speech therapy session. I did a body scan and noticed that my hands were so tightly clenched on the steering wheel that my knuckles were white. I got curious about what was going on with this because after all, I was alone in my car.

It turns out that I was in the future thinking about how much I hated the speech waiting room. While everyone else was sitting nice and quietly, my son would roll on the floor squealing like a pig until his therapist came out for him. I was in the car pre-living this tension filled experience, but I could have been listening to music or enjoying the silence. In my mind, I was pre-experiencing the very situation I was dreading.

But it wasn't just this one incident. When I began tuning in to my body more, I noticed that I was spending a lot of time and energy either pre-experiencing situations or focusing on past experiences that were challenging. I would be doing basic things like washing dishes and notice that my body was in full on fight mode with tense shoulders, clenched jaw and tight stomach like I was bracing for the next hit. I would check in with my thoughts and I was surprised at just how often I was reliving the past or pre-living the future. It's fascinating to realize how those thoughts my Storyteller was creating were manifesting physical tension in my body.

Learning how to question the thoughts and stories the Storyteller has created is an important first step in taking back your power from the Shadow Forces in order to use them more productively to support yourself so you can support your child. If I am in my head thinking about something that happened earlier in the day and my body is tense, I cannot use my mind and body to help in the present moment.

When I notice this is happening, pressing pause and asking questions, like those that follow, can help to process and learn from the previous situation in order to move on.

- *What did that experience/situation teach me?*
- *What can I do to help my future self?*
- *What do I know about my child that I can play with next time?*

When Discomfort Feels Normal

When I first began practicing body scanning, the tension and tightness in my body felt normal even while I was relaxing or doing things that weren't necessarily stressful. Relaxing felt weird. My Storyteller and/or Bodyguard's Warrior energy got very nervous with the idea of relaxing the body. This is totally normal! I practiced by taking deep breaths and reassuring them (my Storyteller and Bodyguard) that all was okay in the present moment.

When you think of what we frequently go through as parents, it's not surprising that we'd be feeling like this, waiting for the next "hit" or preparing for whatever metaphorical balls we have up in the air to drop. This is just the Warrior archetype trying to be helpful AND it is not necessary to live in this constant state of tension. We can acknowledge the uncertainties, stress, anxiety, etc. when they are happening while also not allowing them to seep into times where we could be feeling content.

If you are like me and notice tension and tightness in non-stressful situations, reassure your Bodyguard that you are okay. You can shake it off, yes, literally shake it off (more on that when we talk about the Guardian of Your Heart). Press pause, take several deep breaths, ask those questions I just shared...

- *What did that experience/situation teach me?*
- *What can I do to help my future self out?*
- *What do I know about my child that I can play with next time?*

...and use your senses to get back into the present moment.

The more you notice the connection between your mind and your body, the more energy you will have. You will become adept at questioning your thoughts and relaxing your body, which will give you more energy. You won't be constantly exhausting yourself with your thoughts and storing up negative emotional energy.

Momentary Contentment and Noticing Positive Body Sensations

By the way, learning to listen to your body doesn't have to be only about noticing tension and tightness. It is just as important to learn to recognize your positive body feelings so you can begin to allow yourself to soak in the joy, love and contentment that often pass in a flash and go unnoticed.

When you allow yourself to be in the present moment with your child, even if they are asleep or peering into their iPad's screen, and all is okay in that moment, do a quick body scan for that as well. Notice what it feels like to look at their faces. Notice what it feels like for all to be okay and everyone to be content, without judgmental thoughts.

Here are some common body sensations tied to positive thoughts:

- lightness
- bubbly
- goosebump-y

- expansive
- loose
- relaxed
- open

One of my favorite things to do when my son was young was to reach my hand back while driving somewhere and feel his little foot in my hand. He always took his shoes off and they were usually sweaty little feet, but he's not the snuggliest of people and this simple act made my heart burst with love for him.

These days, I make those heart connections in other ways, often laughing with him about things, like silly internet videos, that I know he will think are funny, give him a kiss on his shoulder or watch him do something he loves to do. I soak it all in and allow myself to feel all of the goose-bumpy feelings as much and as often as possible.

Chapter Ten

Shadow Force #3 - Guardian of Your Heart

This is the part of the hero's journey where you will get to know another aspect of your Warrior archetype, the Guardian of Your Heart. I mentioned this character earlier as the one who swoops in, grabs your heart and tries to protect you by placing you in an emotional lockdown.

Learning that your child is on their own developmental timeline or experiences any challenges that aren't deemed "normal" or "typical" is a shock that is often unexpected, plain and simple. This includes learning, sensory, executive functioning, behavioral and emotional regulation difference challenges, or any type of social difference. I don't know anyone who expects things like this when they are expecting a child.

Few people approach the birth or adoption of their child with the expectation that their child will be confronted with extraordinary, exceptional challenges in processes that are typically taken for granted - challenges in learning and retaining new information, integrating sensory experiences, regulating emotions, controlling behavioral responses, etc.

When I first heard the word autism associated with my son, I remember feeling like the wind was knocked out of me and couldn't breathe. I wanted to cry or yell or punch someone. Fortunately for our pediatrician, I didn't punch her, especially since she was the mom of one of my students (yikes!).

> Please remember this was back in 2004 when knowledge and information about autism was limited, support services weren't what they are today and even if they aren't perfect now, they at least offer some hope.

Everything I felt was pushed down so that I could finish the appointment because I had to be able to get out of her office with some sort of professional composure (again, she was a student's mom), drive home, make dinner and continue being a mom, wife and teacher. My Warrior told me that I needed to be strong and that there wasn't time to process this information or fall apart like I desperately wanted.

The next morning came and I felt like maybe it was all a dream. Once I realized it was very real, all of those emotions came flooding back along with all of the stories of what I was making this new diagnosis mean for our family's future. Yet I couldn't...wouldn't...allow myself to "go there" because breakfast had to be made, the dog needed to go out and I needed to drop my son off at daycare so I could go and teach my third graders.

I thought that if I allowed myself any attention to this newfound information beyond what I needed to do to support him, even for a moment, that I'd get stuck in the big emotions I was feeling and wouldn't be able to function. I did what most people do at times like this and I employed the Guardian of my Heart.

The only thing that my Guardian allowed me to feel was anxiety and a strong desire to make this all go away. As I mentioned earlier, I became extremely controlling in order to keep myself "safe" from the unknown, the what-ifs, my son's meltdowns, the judgment from others and the intensity of emotions within me that were waiting to be felt.

I operated like this for years and discovered that just because you ignore an emotion, it doesn't just go away. The strong emotions I resisted waited patiently for me to be ready. They would attempt to emerge when I would get still to see if it was a good time for them to be processed and released. There never really seemed to be a "good time" to feel strong and intense emotions so this pattern created a resistance to stillness. Yet, stillness, rest and self care is what I desperately needed.

Margaret-ism
Pinballing

As I just mentioned, there were a lot of emotions and thoughts that wanted to be felt and heard, especially when I got still, but since I was nervous and didn't quite know how to process them, I would "pinball" through each and every day. What exactly does that mean? Well, I'd wake up in the morning and just like in a game of pinball (me being the ball), I was shot out into the day, reacting to whatever I bounced off of or whatever caught my attention.

I was taking care of everyone else's wants and needs, without consideration of what I wanted or needed. I did not have any sort of connection with what my intention was for anything other than trying to avoid any sort of tantrum or meltdown. I was strictly operating in "reaction" mode until the end of the day when the game was over and I'd go to bed frustrated that it felt like I didn't accomplish anything.

The thing about pinballing through life is that it feels very busy but it doesn't feel good because there is no intention or purpose behind it. It looked like I was doing lots to take care of my family, but in reality, it was really a way to protect myself from feeling. If I slowed down, the emotions I was avoiding might catch up with me. The negative thoughts might actually be heard and believed.

Pinballing helped keep me numb from this all, and it served me for a while as I could play the role of the exhausted martyr who was always at the mercy of whatever this crazy life threw at me. Although ultimately misguided, pinballing was Warrior energy that temporarily protected me from the overwhelming realization that it was up to me to either embrace or reject the expectations that my Storyteller was creating for our life. When I finally realized pinballing for the protective strategy that it was, I understood that I could create a life that felt better without needing my child to be different. This felt new, weird, big and yes, very scary.

The newfound awareness of my pinballing tendencies initially made me defensive - "This is just who I am and how I do things!" (with a foot stomp like a teenager determined that they know better, which is the Warrior in shadow) - though the more I thought about it, the more I knew deep down that I actually wanted something different.

The noticing of how my pinballing was keeping me from having what I wanted was huge!! While it was normal and comfortable for me to be all over the place, probably also because of undiagnosed attention and executive functioning challenges, that was no longer who I wanted to be or how I wanted to live. I wanted to be more intentional; honestly, the way I was approaching life wasn't working. I wanted to be effective and efficient. I wanted ease and joy. And I wanted these things to exist in the parenting relationship I had with my child.

When I found myself in pinballing mode, I would pause and check in with my intention for that moment. From there, I gave that my attention which meant things got done or resolved and I felt more content.

Emotional Lockdown

Turns out that a lot of parents on this hero's journey in parenting fear that feeling the intense emotions surrounding an unexpected twist in their parenting life will render them unable to function. However, the opposite ends up being true. Not allowing yourself to process your emotions actually leads to exhaustion.

I don't want you to be on "emotional lockdown" any longer and want to support you in building a different relationship with your own personal Guardian of your Heart. There are ways to experience and release emotions in safe and healthy ways, using them as indicators for what you are wanting and/or needing in order to parent in a way that feels better. I will be going into this in greater detail later on, but wanted to introduce this concept as it is an extremely common thing for parents to do when given a diagnosis or label.

While this is sometimes necessary in order to function after receiving some unexpected or startling information, when your Guardian acts overprotective, it becomes a Shadow Force. It is trying to keep you safe from the intensity of the emotions that come from all of the unexpecteds during the Hero's Journey in Parenting, but in doing this, it blocks you from feeling *any* emotion...including ease, joy and contentment.

Warning! Relieving your Guardian of all of the duties it has placed upon itself is most likely to send you running back to the threshold, or closing this book. Please don't!! I get this 100% because this is exactly what I wanted to do when I began this process. Over time, I built a relationship with the normal human emotions that I had been storing and resisting for years. Doing this allowed my Guardian to relax a bit so that I could not only release emotions I had been avoiding, but also learn how these emotions were trying to support me in the present moment.

Before I understood this, if I had even a sliver of a thought about allowing myself to get curious about my stored emotions, my Guardian took over with more conviction than ever. My Warrior was very adamant about all of the dangers I would be exposed to if I were to open up that vault where it had been keeping my heart.

The Guardian teamed up with my Storyteller creating lots of stories about what would happen if I felt emotions. "I would be vulnerable." "It would be too intense." "I'm going to get stuck in them." "I need to be 'strong' for my child."

Situations that brought attention to his challenges or how he was different from his chronological peers (whether behaviorally, socially or academically) brought waves of emotions to the surface, but I pushed them down. Meetings with school professionals, neuro-psychologists or doctors left me with a clenched jaw, a tight stomach and a heavy heart. This was my child, my baby, they were talking about!

I wanted to be reminded of what an amazing child he actually was, focus on the things that he was able to do, celebrate the growth and progress that he was making, even if it was on his own developmental timeline!

> I eventually learned that I needed to do those things myself and not rely on others to do them for me.

I don't know anyone who wants to feel strong, uncomfortable emotions. My Guardian and Storyteller were telling me very convincing stories in order to protect my ego from feeling inadequate. However, when I began to examine those stories and look at my emotions, I realized what I had been believing all along – that my son wasn't going to be happy until x, y or z happened or that I wasn't a good parent – weren't true...at all!

Despite what I feared, I actually became much stronger by allowing myself to be honest and acknowledge the emotions I was feeling, but had been repressing. Emotions are energy in motion. They are meant to support us; that is their purpose. Building a new relationship with them creates a shift from being at their mercy to recognizing the importance of allowing healthy processing and the ability to release them.

The simple fact was that I was already thinking and feeling these things. As I shared previously, my feelings and thoughts about the past, present and future created energy and physical responses in the body that felt like events that were happening in real time.

Undercurrent of Energy

"Please take responsibility for the
energy you bring into this space."

Jill Bolte Taylor in "Stroke of Insight"

Emotions create energy and don't simply go away when they aren't acknowledged. They get stored in the body, almost like there is an imaginary PVC pipe inside of you that they get shoved into. This leads to an "undercurrent of energy" that is woven into everything you do and can keep you from being in alignment with how you actually want to feel and show up in your life. Awareness of this is important for us as parents because everyone can pick up on it...especially our children.

Sometimes the undercurrent of energy is warm, loving, open and accepting, which feels amazing to be around, and is usually the result of a person taking care of their needs so that they are clear and aware of what they are doing and feeling.

Sometimes this energy feels funky or dissonant and shows up in interactions as resentment, frustration or annoyance. Think about times when someone has asked you how you are doing and you respond with a sharp, "Fine." Chances are they picked up on the undercurrent of energy you were putting out and were either trying to figure out what was going on or exited the situation quickly.

You may notice that while you are on the Hero's Journey in Parenting, the "undercurrent of energy" is fueled by sadness, grief, anger or confusion. Your Storyteller works on crafting stories about how the other people in your life "should" behave, respond and treat you. With your Warrior activated and ready to defend, your Battle Ready Bodyguard clamps down, leaving your body feeling tense and tight. This stance is in opposition to the open and loving person that you want to be with those you hold dear.

What does this look like?

You may have the intention and desire to make dinner for your family in order to nourish and show your love for them. In reality, you are exhausted after a tough day of whatever life and parenting has thrown your way. You may have had a tough conversation with a teacher about how your child is doing in class and are shoving down the feelings of sadness, frustration, confusion, etc. because you needed to finish your work day.

You start to feel resentment and frustration because nobody has helped, people are doing whatever they want to do (most likely focused on their screens) and when dinner is ready, you set down the plates and sigh. You inhale your food while totally in your head as your Storyteller is busy crafting thoughts around how annoying and entitled these people are and how they should help more.

They should see how tired I am after a long day. Would it be too much to ask for someone to offer a hand without being asked or told? They should acknowledge that I do everything for them and how much I would appreciate even the smallest gesture of gratitude or assistance.

You may have the intention and desire to have a wonderful, laid back family vacation. Reality looks more like you being the one who is taking care of everything, remembering all that needs to be done, arranged, packed and charged. You do this because you have all of their wants and needs on your metaphorical radar screen in order to do what needs to be done to avoid meltdowns, tantrums and complaining. (We will be exploring meltdowns and tantrums in a later section.)

You do all of this and then when it's time to leave, someone makes a comment about how you are never ready on time. You glare at them, making a snarky comment under your breath about how it must be nice to just pack one's own bag and be ready in five minutes.

> Just because you can do something or are good at it, doesn't mean you have to do it. If you choose to do it because it'll make you feel better, that brings a totally different energy! If it would feel better to pass on some responsibility to others, use the TIANT Process I'll be sharing later on and take some time to think about what that could look like in order to feel confident knowing things are still getting done.

Get Curious!

The way out of the murky undercurrent of energy is something we have access to at all times and that is the ability to tap into curiosity. The more curious you get, the more you will begin to notice your personal "tells." For me, I notice my tone as it gets more snarky and sharp. My stomach feels tight and my energy feels like a volcano bubbling. This is simply my Battle Ready Bodyguard activating, attempting to set boundaries, though going about it in shadowy ways.

These scenarios - fictitious of course as nobody in my life would ever do anything like that (ha!) - are meant to show what happens when you don't take care of yourself and ask for what you want and need from those around you. Not asking for what you need because you are having a hard time relinquishing control creates an undercurrent of energy that is the opposite of what you are actually wanting to feel, experience and convey.

If you notice that your undercurrent of energy is more tension filled than you would like, asking yourself the basic questions, *"What is causing me tension?"* and *"What is my intention right now?"* can create a perspective shift in order to get clarity around what you are wanting...even if what you want is to make dinner AND have someone offer to help.

Most likely what you really want isn't just help. You want that empathy piece from the other person that lets them see and understand that you are feeling a bit put upon and makes them WANT to help you. Which is not to say that learning to ask for the help you want is not a valuable skill. It certainly is. But so is asking people to be a little more sensitive to your needs so that you don't have to always ask when you want help.

From there, you can zoom out in order to task your Storyteller with being curious about what actually needs to happen in order to take care of your wants/needs. You might also ask for support while keeping in mind what is realistic and doable for all involved. Knowing what you want is one thing but having a better understanding of the attention that is needed and/or wanted is what helps create a completely different undercurrent of energy, one that feels clear and in alignment with words and actions.

Once you've gotten clarity around what is possible, you can be more clear and direct about what you want from yourself, the experience and others. This process allows your Monarch/Elder archetype to direct your Warrior in a more helpful and productive fashion.

Example:

One Sunday morning, years ago, I was busy scrubbing the daylight out of some dirty pots and pans when I realized that my Battle Ready Bodyguard had allowed some murky emotions to pop up---I was feeling annoyed and resentful. So I checked in with the thoughts that my Storyteller was busy creating. When I did this, I noticed that I was annoyed with my husband because when I looked over into our living room, I saw this ideal morning playing out that I was not a part of. There was a fire in the fireplace because it was cold and gray outside and he was sitting there reading the New Yorker, with our dog snuggled against him and our son playing contentedly with his marble coaster.

*Wasn't I always craving cozy mornings like this?
Yes and it turned out that I wanted to be part of
that scene, relaxing rather than cleaning the kitchen!
I then got curious about why I was annoyed with
my husband since he wasn't doing anything wrong.
I realized that I was jealous of him doing what he
wanted and actually enjoying the morning. I was
totally in my head "should-ing" on him!*

- *He should notice that I'm still cleaning.*
- *He should come in and help me.*
- *He should know that I'd love to be relaxing
  too, rather than cleaning.*

*This awareness of my thoughts and all of the
"should-ing" that was taking place cracked me up
and I realized some important things about this
scenario. The first was that I had chosen to start
cleaning the kitchen. He didn't care about a clean
kitchen at that moment and is always more than
willing to clean things up with me.*

*The second realization rocked my world. I had
choices! I could choose to stop cleaning and go relax.
I could choose to continue cleaning knowing I decided
to do this and then afterwards, relax. I could also
choose to ask for help.*

*The funny thing is that I chose to continue cleaning
but my energy totally changed from being jealous*

and resentful to feeling content with my choice. I knew I was almost done and that it would feel good to be done with it. I also got out of my head and enjoyed the music that was playing along with the feeling of love and contentment knowing my family was safe, sound and happy on a lovely Sunday morning.

The next time you notice that your undercurrent of energy is annoyance or frustration, ask yourself...

What am I actually annoyed or frustrated about?

As mentioned before, this question will give you insights into what you are wanting or needing help with so that you can get curious about what this looks like in your life, in that situation.

This may involve relinquishing some control and allowing things to be a little messy or to be done differently than you may typically do them. But realizing that what you are doing is a consequence of your choice changes everything---your energy, your feelings, your experience---because now you have taken ownership of not only your behavior, but also of the CHOICE you made to engage in that behavior. Choosing to do things can change everything - your energy, your feelings, your experience, etc. - as it is YOUR choice.

There are times when I have the time, energy and patience to have my son do something new or challenging, and other times the situation might be time sensitive and I choose to do it for him. Recognizing and acknowledging this will create an undercurrent of energy that feels aligned and clear for everyone and that feels so much better!

The reality is that you are feeling normal human emotions. When you don't allow yourself to process and release these emotions, they build up, along with the stories your Storyteller concocts and the tensions they trigger within you. And whether you realize it or not, these weighty emotions are there inside you, shaping your thoughts, feelings and actions, until you allow yourself to feel them.

> If they feel too big, get professional help to support you in processing and releasing them. While I am not a therapist, psychologist or psychiatrist, I've included some specific strategies for each specific emotion that I found to be helpful in my journey.

As much as I wanted to resist feeling my own emotions, I came to learn that it was crucial if I wanted to have more peace, ease and joy in my life. It was exhausting to stay busy and shoving them down, pretending like I was "fine" worked okay until something irritated me. When that happened, small bits of emotion would seep out in the form of passive aggressive remarks or a snarkiness to my tone.

I felt controlling, tight and heavy. None of this was intentional and my son and husband would ask me why I said something in the way that I did or why I was acting in a defensive manner. It annoyed me when they inquired and they were onto something I didn't even realize - I was avoiding feeling emotions.

This avoidance lasted until I was at a coaching retreat with Martha Beck and Koelle Simpson (two of my own coaches and mentors) where horses were used as part of the coaching process. I was in the round pen with a horse who had no harness. I had no way to control him or force him to do anything. The coaches instructed us to have an intention for what we wanted before we entered the pen and while with the horse, try different things to make it happen.

> This is a similar coaching exercise as the one match fire making task I described earlier. The fire making task gave me insight into how I approach things. The round pen horse experience offered the same insight, but with the added benefit of opening my eyes as to how I approach relationships with other living things.

Well, my horse wasn't doing anything I wanted it to do despite all of the energy I was putting into trying to get something "right" and make something happen. My horse wasn't doing any of the things that the other horses did when they were in the round pen with their people. This all felt incredibly familiar and prompted the coaching question, "Where else does this show up in your life?" Everywhere!!

My thoughts went to things like...

- *Why can't my son sit nice and still in the waiting room like the other kids?*

- *Why can't I get him to talk?*
- *Why can't I potty train him?*

When my coach asked what I was thinking, I responded that I felt just like I did parenting my son. Regardless of what I tried that I had seen other people do, nothing worked.

Because I was in a safe environment where I trusted the process and my coaches, my Guardian of the Heart was disarmed. I left the round pen, went around the corner and began to sob hysterically. Shortly afterwards, I felt extremely vulnerable. My Warrior jumped right back into action, employing the Storyteller, Bodyguard and Guardian to take control and shove those feelings and thoughts back down to where they had been residing all of those years.

Fortunately, I was at a coaching retreat and this sort of reaction was nothing new for the facilitators. It was an important part of the process. Once again, I was faced with two choices – stay exactly where I was, exhausted from avoiding emotions, or take that step towards the unknown and trust that all would be okay.

I was scared as hell am here to tell you that I was able to convince the Guardian of my Heart to stand back. I slowly and intentionally opened the vault, felt the feelings and am still here to talk about it.

Before this next section on Opening the Vault, it is imperative for me to again express the significance of having some sort of support in place, whether it is a therapist, psychologist, psychiatrist or experienced coach, especially if you have experienced trauma in your life. If you have been repressing emotions as a defensive and protective mechanism, there is a reason, so having a professional who can help you feel safe and supported while knowing how to guide you through them is key. My intention is to share what helped me to find hope and release what was keeping me stuck. I did not do this on my own. I had support from my coaches to help me through this.

Opening the Vault

I went back to my hotel room and began what is now one of my favorite coaching strategies for opening the vault to process and release – I wrote letters. I wrote letters to myself and to my son that I would burn the next day. At first it was controlled and filtered and then something shifted and as I allowed myself to write without judgment or fear. It all came pouring out. Every single emotion seemed to be pushing for its expression.

I felt sadness.

I felt anger.

I felt grief.

I felt confusion.

I felt guilt and shame.

I felt it all. I sat on the bed and let it go. I sobbed and sobbed. The sobbing usually lasted about 90 seconds (which I've since learned is the typical amount of time it takes to release an emotion when we have stopped resisting them) and then it subsided for a short time before the next wave of stored emotion would come.

Without resisting, I continued to let the process unfold, letting go. Eventually, there wasn't anything left to feel at that time. That night, I slept very soundly and while I woke up with puffy eyes, I also woke up feeling some new feelings – relief, inspiration and hope!

If you can relate to any of this, I strongly encourage you to find support, setting yourself up so that you feel as safe as possible. Once I had processed and released a lot of the deep emotions I had been repressing under the guidance of my coaches, I began to feel more comfortable about processing and releasing them on my own.

There was still the old pattern of nervousness about getting stuck in the muck of suck. Because of this, if I noticed there was an emotion that wanted to be felt but couldn't process and release in the moment that the incident took place, I could tuck it away temporarily until I did have time to explore what was going on.

When there was time, I went into that experience with a great deal of intention. I chose a time and place where I could be alone or call a trusted person who would listen without judgment. I set parameters around how long the process and release session would be by setting my timer for 5 -10 minutes, knowing that when the timer went off, I could take a deep breath and check in with how I was doing. Was I feeling okay? Was I feeling like it was too much? If it was too much, I would schedule a session with my coach. If I was feeling okay but needed to move on with my day, I could close the door on the vault until the next time.

> This is a great way to utilize the Warrior energy in order to set some boundaries so that my Storyteller could relax a bit, not offering all sorts of unhelpful thoughts and stories.

Allow whatever wants to be expressed without judgment. When I think about what this was like for me, it was very much like the scene in the movie "Steel Magnolias" where Sally Fields' character is in the cemetery grieving for her daughter. She experiences all of the emotions and just lets them fly going from grief to anger to guilt to sadness to laughter (I'm probably dating myself with this movie so if you haven't seen it, here is a link to a YouTube clip - https://www.youtube.com/watch?v=iZx1W6cHw-g).

My initial fears around feeling emotions, that I would get stuck and/or be weakened by allowing them, were proven false. I became much stronger by allowing myself to be honest and acknowledge what I was feeling. I was no longer spending my energy running away from my emotions. My undercurrent of energy became healthy and powerful. I faced my feelings with courage and learned the messages each of them had for me. I began viewing them like a team of friends who only want the best for me. The more I got used to allowing them, the faster I could feel and cycle through them.

You may label emotions as good or bad as I did, but I have learned that they are all trying to help us process whatever is going on. I love the Pixar movie "Inside Out" because it illustrates this beautifully, with each emotion sitting at the control panel and impacting responses based on whatever was going on. Acknowledging that all emotions are okay, even anger, helped me build a new relationship with them. I found ways to release the stored up sadness, grief, fear and anger and also learned what to do with emotions as they emerged in the present moment.

> Karla McLaren wrote a wonderful book called *Language of Emotions* if you'd like to learn more.

The most helpful way I have found to connect with my emotions when I notice tension is to ask...

- *What is it that I am feeling?*
- *How is it trying to help or support me?*

If you do this, you might be surprised by what shows up. Like the "Steel Magnolias" scene, it could be a medley of emotions all tangled up in one thought or situation. No judgment. No need to narrow them down. Simply get curious about how they are trying to help you.

It can also be helpful to find a quiet place, get still and see what emerges. This is something I have been playing with.

As soon as I get still, the emotion is right there. These days it usually takes about five minutes to release it and then I can go back to what I was doing.

Now, let's wander a bit together to get perspective about what is actually going on and learn some ways that you can process your stored up emotions.

Dealing with the Emotions Released- Anger

Anger can be thought of as a response to three broad categories of perceived threat - threats to our safety, threats to our control and threats to our self-value. Understanding that anger is a response to a perceived threat helps explain why anger is typically described as a secondary emotion, like confusion, frustration, annoyance, fear, hurt, embarrassment, shame, guilt, etc. It is those primary emotions that fuel anger.

- Threats to our safety show up through fear, confusion, vulnerability, etc.
- Threats to our control are felt as frustration, annoyance and helplessness.
- Threats to our self-value make us feel ashamed, annoyed, guilty, embarrassed, etc.

This is also helpful to consider and be curious about when your child is feeling strong emotions. What might they feel is threatening them? Safety? Control? Self-value? Knowing there is more going on than behaviors, actions, reactions can allow for very different approaches and conversations with those on your child's team.

Thinking about anger this way has a number of benefits for people who are trying to determine the source of their anger and manage their response to it. So, when they are feeling angry, questions they might ask themselves would include:

- *Is the situation that's making me angry threatening my safety (or the safety of someone I care about), my sense of control or my self-value?*
- *What primary emotion related to that threat is fueling my anger (Am I frustrated? Annoyed? Embarrassed? Confused? Afraid?)*

Understanding that anger is a response to a perceived threat helps explain why two people, experiencing the same situation, respond differently. Someone with higher control needs will be more sensitive to potential threats to their control. Someone with a more fragile sense of their competence in some domain will be more sensitive to potential threats to their self-value. This is good to know because if you realize that most of your anger is coming from perceived threats to your sense of control, the work you need to do to manage that will be different than if most of your anger is coming from perceived threats to your self-worth. (Again, good to know in order to best support your child and what their needs might be.)

In parenting, anger can happen when a boundary has been crossed by someone's words or actions - like someone making an unkind comment or giving a dirty look directed at your child. It can also happen when the boundary of expectations has been challenged or broken - like getting a diagnosis or label about your child. Both of these boundary crossings are perceived threats to the safety of my family, my sense of control and my self-value as a parent and brought up questions like:

- What would the future be like for us?
- Would our marriage make it?
- Would we be able to care for him in the way he would need?
- Would I be a good mom for him, the mom he deserved?
- What would the future be like for him?
- Would he be safe in an often unkind world?
- Would he be able to receive services that would support him in achieving his highest potential?

When I allowed myself to become curious about what I was actually feeling with regards to my son's diagnosis, there was a lot of anger around not being able to choose this journey. I was frustrated and annoyed that the choice had been made for me. I had been pushed over the threshold into a life I knew nothing about which made me feel confused and inadequate. As a former teacher, I felt embarrassment and guilt because I didn't know more about how best to support him in those early days.

Once I realized that anger was present, I got scared. It was an emotion that I feared connecting with because despite feeling it, I listened to my Storyteller's thoughts such as, "What kind of mother am I if I feel angry?" I worried that allowing it would unleash a temper I knew all too well from my childhood and had been trying to avoid like the plague.

Anger is one of the most common emotions for parents and it also brings up the most shame and guilt. It is an emotion that people often like to leapfrog right over because they feel like it is not okay to feel angry about the situation that they are in and yet, when it seeps out, all sorts of "should-ing" happens around this like...

- *I shouldn't have been upset.*
- *I shouldn't have yelled.*
- *I should have done xyz.*
- *I should have been calm.*

This "should-ing" usually follows a string of events where there is not enough self-care or kids are dysregulated, pushing buttons, being annoying (as kids will be from time to time) or are unable to do what we'd like them to do.

This last one might bring up shame and guilt AND when I got honest with myself, there were times I was angry that my son couldn't do what I wanted him to do. This was 100% my stuff and had nothing to do with him. Rather than beating myself up, it gave me an opportunity to find ways to meet him where he was so that I could support him while also supporting myself during those situations.

When people don't recognize the anger building and learn to release it in healthy ways, it seeps out in shadowy ways, usually towards those we are closest to. When I say "shadowy" I mean things like sarcasm, negative tones, harsh language, resentment, passive aggressiveness or erupting with strong emotions unexpectedly, often unrelated to what is happening in the present moment.

Something that shocked me to realize was that I could be one who allowed the boundary to be crossed. All of those times when I said "Sure!" but really wanted to say "No." All of those times that I didn't check in with my intention and handed over decision making power to others despite having clear wants and needs. This was all good to know so I could come up with strategies to allow myself time to think.

- *I need to check my calendar.*
- *Let me think on this before I commit.*

Having things like this to say when feeling pressured helped me to give myself the boundaries I needed, mainly time and space to think, in order to make decisions that were best for me.

Once you have some clarity around what is causing the anger, get curious about what you can do to support yourself based on what you've learned. Does the anger feel huge and out of control? If so, consult with a professional to help you. I've been on the receiving end of that kind of anger and wish that the person who exploded on me physically and verbally would have gotten some sort of professional help.

If not, ask yourself what would feel really good as a way of releasing it. (That might sound weird but it can help to determine if it is something that needs to be expressed verbally or released physically in safe and healthy ways of course.)

Do you feel the need to express something?

If so...

- Get in your car and yell! Go in your garage or find an empty parking lot and say everything you'd like to say as though you are yelling at the person you are angry at.
- Write a letter allowing whatever wants to come out without filter or judgment and say whatever wants to be expressed and then burn it. This is important because it is just for you and is not for anyone else to find.
- Call a trusted person and consciously complain or vent without them trying to fix things, problem solve or jump on the bandwagon.

> I have had times where I was so angry about a situation I wanted to scream at the top of my lungs at a person. I've actually done it and it didn't feel better because the person didn't respond the way I wanted or needed to have the situation resolved.

Do you feel the need to physically release it? Get curious about what is realistic in your life that could serve the purpose of releasing that fight energy. Here are some ideas...

- Use a plastic bat and gather up pillows in a comforter and hit the pile of fluff.
- Slam a medicine ball (the soft leather kind as the rubber kind can bounce up and hit you in the face - speaking from personal experience with this one - ha!!).
- Sign up for a kickboxing class.
- Hit a tennis ball as hard as you can.
- Yell or scream while alone in your car especially if you notice a tightness in your throat and feel like you are not being heard or understood (sharing this again as it is one of my favorites!)
- Do something physical while holding the intention of releasing the anger you have about the situation until you feel the strong emotional energy is gone.

This is another one of those times when the emotion usually dissipates in 90 seconds. Once the feeling isn't so intense, there is usually a good deal of clarity around how to proceed, what changes you need to make (if anything), what you need to communicate and how best to communicate it.

If I allow myself to do this in a safe and healthy way — like screaming in my car alone — I can release that hot anger. Then, when I express myself later to the person, some anger may still be present, but it isn't infused with the same intensity of strong emotion. Letting some air out of my anger and calming my response usually helps the other person be more willing to hear me and we can then work together to find a resolution.

Start getting curious about how anger typically looks, sounds or feels for you so that you can pause and figure out what you are wanting or needing in order to release it. Notice what boundaries were crossed, even if it was yourself who crossed them. Use that information to get clear about what attention you can give to support yourself, and others, in the future.

Doing so helped me to shift from avoiding feeling anger, yet having an "undercurrent of energy" fueled by it, to allowing myself to learn from it. This always helps me cycle through it faster, and it can help you as well.

Dealing with the Emotions Released-Sadness

When I began to explore the emotion of sadness, I discovered how to allow myself to experience what I was feeling deep down when things didn't go the way that I wanted rather than putting on my "fine" face.

Sadness shows up when the reality of our situation does not match our expectations, and/or we feel like we have lost something or we actually have lost something. At first my sadness felt like it would be too big and too much to feel. I was afraid I would get stuck in my grief, I would become depressed and it would be tough to do anything for my son. What I didn't realize back then was that even though I was resisting feeling sad, the "undercurrent of sad energy" was with me even when I was with my child trying to be happy.

Feeling sad or disappointed is normal!! Recognizing what is causing the sadness helps you care for yourself so that you can release that emotional energy in order to accept, appreciate and feel gratitude for the life that you have.

When something happens that creates sadness, give yourself some time and space to feel the feelings with intention. Putting words to it can help you ask for what you are wanting or needing from yourself and/or those around you. For example – I wasn't expecting this and I need 5 minutes to feel sad or disappointed about this.

From there, it is helpful to ask yourself the question...

What am I making this mean?

This one question can lead to all sorts of juicy thoughts and stories created by your Storyteller and are perfect for Byron Katie's Inquiry Process "The Work."

I remember feeling really sad while at the playground because my son was always swinging alone or doing things by himself, while other moms huddled in groups chatting away happily while their children ran around together. I would follow him because he was anxious about me getting lost. I didn't mind this at first but after a while, I was sad that he wasn't playing with other kids.

I noticed my sadness and got curious. This was an important awareness for me! I came out of my thought fog and looked at him. He was swinging on the swing, shoes kicked off, with THE BIGGEST smile on his face. He couldn't have cared less and was not bothered one bit by playing alone while his mom was nearby. He probably didn't even feel alone since I was there! This was all my stuff, not his. I was sad, he was not.

I was sad because I had expectations to be in the group of chatting moms. I wanted friends to schedule playdates with and can think back to early "Mommy and Me" type classes where the other moms children would be following along, sitting in their laps clapping, using instruments and singing songs while mine ran around finding things he found more interesting. I would watch those moms chat and laugh and at the end, they would exchange phone numbers in order to set up playdates. I wasn't chatting with anyone because I followed him around to keep him safe and off of the more interesting items that we were told weren't for him. Nobody asked for my number.

I wanted people to not look at me like we had the plague when I mentioned that he wasn't speaking yet or that he was autistic. I felt very alone and just wanted to have a mom friend.

> This was a major source of my intention and motivation for the "Parenting the Child You Didn't Expect While You Were Expecting" tele-courses that I created as I didn't want other moms out there feeling as alone as I did.

After that wake-up call at the playground, shifting my expectations for those visits and taking care of myself, I was really able to soak in that what brought him joy looked different.

I was making it mean that I could only be happy if he was happily playing with other kids. I was making it mean that I was missing out on something. Not true!! I did "The Work" on my Storyteller's thoughts and as I got more clear about my intentions for parenting my child, I began shifting perspectives which led me to so much more ease, peace and joy!

If you can relate to the scenarios I described above and are feeling sadness, please know you are not alone.

What can you do to release the sadness?

- Give yourself time and space to curl up and cry while wrapped in a blanket.

- Write a loving letter to yourself acknowledging all that you've been through and burn it.
- Write a loving letter to your child and burn it.
- With intention, have a little pity party for yourself to acknowledge the truth that things not going as expected does make you sad. Pretending things are "fine" will just create more dissonance, almost like your essential self will say, "Ummmm...are you not seeing what I'm seeing?"

For these ideas, I recommend setting a timer before you begin so that you know that there is a beginning and an end to your session. Also, acknowledge the times when you are "stuck in the muck of suck" or playing the victim/martyr of the situation. For me, this recognition helps me see what is actually going on which helps me move through it faster.

Dealing with the Emotions Released- Fear

The oldest and strongest emotion of mankind is fear, and the oldest and strongest kind of fear is fear of the unknown.

H. P. Lovecraft

Fear is a very common emotion when parenting a child who is on their own developmental timeline because it is filled with the unknown. The Storyteller is always quick to bring up fears based on past experiences and how any decisions you make could impact your child. Fears of the present moment and doubts about whether or not you are doing enough as a parent or being a good enough parent, and fears of the future and what that will be like for the child.

Fear is that part of our brain that convinces us that worry is helpful, that at least by worrying, we are doing something that feels productive. Fear also confronts the reality that we are not in control. Fear is just the Storyteller trying to protect you, even if it does so in a misguided way, in order to prepare you for the worst.

Fear freaks the crap out of the Warrior and triggers the part of our brain that is wired to help us survive. We either try to fight it or get away from it. Again, most of the time, the things we fear are those things that are out of our control. Getting stuck in fear only works to suck our energy and our ability to use energy and attention in helpful ways or even to enjoy the present moment.

Asking yourself the simple, yet powerful, question...

What am I worried about?

...can give you some insight into where your fear is coming from.

When you are worried, most of the time your Storyteller is busy reminding you about something that has already happened, replaying it over and over in your mind, thinking about what should have been done or said.

Your Storyteller may also be crafting stories about what might happen in the future and what you could say or do or how your child might react or respond.

| School tends to bring this up for a lot of parents.

Fear-based thoughts about the past and/or the future, real or imagined, are ultimately counterproductive since the outcomes in both situations are beyond your control. You cannot do anything about them regardless of how convincing your Storyteller is. The reality is that the only moment you have any influence over is the present moment. You can use what you know about yourself and your child to try and set yourselves up for success, or at least manage challenging situations, but you cannot control anyone.

Learning to stay in the present moment and get curious by putting the creativity of your Storyteller to work about your fear, will help you respond to any situation in a way that is most aligned with your intention.

This is easier said than done and this is what I consider to be true meditation: the ability to be in the presence of someone experiencing discomfort...even yourself...and not try to force things to be different from what they are. Rather, use curiosity to see what you can influence or do to support those experiencing the discomfort.

This is where noticing and awareness come into play. The ability to check in with yourself, your thoughts and your body with the question...

What is actually going on?

...in order to get curious about what is actually going on and what you are actually feeling, allows for greater connection with ourselves and our children.

What can you do when the emotion you are feeling is fear?

- You can tap into curiosity around what and where the fear is coming from. Is it something happening in real time, like a child running out into the street? Or is it reliving or pre-living from a "What if?" perspective. Most fear is the latter, though I've certainly had my times of fearing for my child's safety as he slipped out of my hand in a busy parking lot.

- Get curious about how it might be serving or helping you. Fear is just the Storyteller trying to protect you in order to prepare you for the worst. Thank it for trying to be helpful and then let it go with a deep breath and little shake.

Here are some of my favorite strategies...

- Put words to it, verbally or in writing. One of the things I do when I'm worried or fearful is to tell my worry doll. I have these little dolls that someone gave me years ago and their job is to worry for me so I don't have to. I also use them with my son and it really helps him to close the loop on things he is worried about so he can move on.

- Another thing I do is to ask someone to worry for me. Doing this creates some energetic distance between my thoughts and stories and the reality of the present moment. Pick someone who isn't actually going to worry about it! I frequently get texts and emails from clients asking me to worry about school meetings, family gatherings, camp tryouts and new playdates.

- Draw a picture of your fear. This is one of my dear friend Katie's favorite things to do as her fears are quite funny when she does this and it helps take the power and charge out of them. One example was her drawing of everything that the ideal mom would be doing and it quickly became obvious that all the expectations and fears she was putting on herself were beyond doable.

- Write out all of the "and then" situations you can think of and reread them with the perspective that in the present moment, you have NO idea what the future holds AND you cannot control what happens. It can be quite comical and will shine a light on how dramatic and creative our Storyteller can be creating scary stories about what might happen.

- Just like with anger, sometimes I feel the need to scream in my car after a scare.
- I imagine that my body is like a french press coffee maker, plunging the unnecessary energy back into the ground and out of my body. (This is a Margaret-ism that I will describe in greater detail shortly.)
- I shake my body as though I'm shaking the energy off of me.

By the way, shaking off energy created by fear and anger is totally natural! Animals do this all of the time, watch them. They either shake or yawn. While we humans with our creative brains hold onto emotional energy through the stories and thoughts we have about things, animals do not. Once the actual fearful experience has passed, they no longer need the fight or flight energy to survive and they get on with whatever they are doing in the present moment. It does nothing to support their survival to hold onto it.

Example:

A few years ago I was co-leading a day retreat at HorseLink and we got to see first hand what shaking off fear-based energy looks like with an animal.

HorseLink is a wonderful place where retired show horses go. The owner of the HorseLink Foundation, Julie Puentes, provides land and care for them, while using them to support coaching and healing for those experiencing PTSD, trauma and things like navigating unexpecteds in parenting.

We were about to start a grooming exercise in order for our clients to connect with these beautiful animals by brushing them, when one of Julie's beloved horses, Big Head Todd, ducked his head under his harness line. When he tried to raise his head, realized he was stuck. He got agitated and Julie knew she needed to get him out of his harness or he'd hurt himself.

She calmly went to him, speaking gently while also being careful knowing she could also get hurt. She was able to unbuckle the harness and backed away so he could get out of it. He did and then ran around the pen for a short while before stopping and shaking a big full body shake. After that, he found a little patch of grass and began eating, which I've been told means he feels comfortable and safe.

It was a scary thing to watch and even more so for Julie to experience with a horse she has had since it was born AND it was perfect because we got to witness the importance of staying calm. We also saw that even though he was scared, he shook it off and then went about his day without carrying around any stories about it.

We joked about how silly it would be if later on we saw him talking to another horse, Fallon, recounting the story of how he got stuck, almost died and how scared he was...like we would probably do. This is why it is important to notice the stories our Storyteller is creating and check in on whether or not they are helping us or keeping us stuck in them.

Margaret-ism
French Press Energy Release Method

As someone who has been playing with noticing when fear, anxiety, control and anger pop up in my body and also how to consciously and intentionally release that energy from my body, particularly energy and emotion that is not mine, I got a very powerful image one day of what this actually looked like - a french press coffee maker!

Quite often, we can hold onto energy and emotion that is not serving us, mainly when we get stuck in the stories, thoughts and beliefs about how things "should" or "shouldn't" have been. It may feel like once you notice this that you "should" just get over it and move on. I've found that it's not always that easy and so I like to have this tool to help me separate and release intentionally.

Other times, we can take on other people's "stuff" as we talk with them, listen to the challenges and annoyances that they may have. Think back to a time where you were talking with a friend or family member about something stressful that they were experiencing and once home, you notice that you are still thinking about their stressful situation and are short and snappy with your family members. If so, you probably took on their stress and emotion.

It's one thing to be empathetic and supportive but it is not helpful to literally take on their emotions. When this happens, it is helpful to check in with yourself to see if what you are feeling is yours or if it belongs to someone else. If it is yours, get curious about what is actually going on and utilize some of the strategies to help you release the emotion in safe and healthy ways.

Bringing to mind the way a french press coffee maker works could help you release what is not serving you. If you are not familiar with this, you place ground coffee into the pot, fill it with boiling water, let it steep and then slowly plunge down to separate the grounds from the liquid that is now coffee. Imagine that the coffee grounds are the thoughts, stories and emotions and while I believe that there is always something to learn or practice, separating from the thoughts and stories can help one move forward without the sludge.

When I do this, I stand with my feet firmly on the ground, take some deep breaths to get into my body and out of my head, and then imagine slowly plunging any tension, stories, thoughts or emotion that is not necessary down through my feet into the ground in order to get clarity around what matters and can help me move forward. Sometimes I have to plunge a couple of times in order to feel like I've released it all…and that's okay.

Allowing yourself to connect with your emotions will help you to start building a different, more healthy relationship with them. You can begin simply by asking yourself what you are feeling and then inquire as to how the emotion or emotions you are feeling are trying to help you.

You might be surprised by what shows up, especially if there is an emotion underneath another emotion. Your primary emotion might be anger at your child's teacher. But when you start exploring a little more, there is also fear...fear for your child's future, fear for how your child feels while they are in school or fear of "what if" scenarios that could create challenging changes for you all.

Do not judge any of what you are feeling as each emotion just wants to help us process and release. Give yourself permission to just be with them and let them do their thing and you might notice that their intensity comes and goes in 90 second waves. The more you resist feeling them, the more they will persist as they become fueled by the thoughts and stories your Storyteller creates.

If in sharing my experiences about how I learned to recognize and release unhelpful emotions I have implied that this process was easy for me, let me assure you that it was NOT! It took some time for me to trust this. I can now say that when I do, it is incredibly freeing and I move through them more quickly. When I am honest with myself and taking care of my own emotions, this allows me to be a better mom for my son.

> I have not forgotten about joy. There is a whole chapter later on in the book devoted to it so if you'd like to skip ahead to check that out, go for it!!

Chapter Eleven

The Importance of Stillness

As I previously mentioned, the ability to press pause is something that can be incredibly helpful in understanding your Storyteller, your Battle Ready Bodyguard and the Guardian of Your Heart. Allowing yourself to practice stillness, even in the smallest of doses, is like the Disney FastPass (or now the Lightning Lane, Genie Pass or perhaps something else these days!) to see how each of these characters show up in your life.

My first experience with the practice of stillness came after reading "The Joy Diet" by Martha Beck. I wanted joy again and this seemed like a great place to start. The first exercise in this book was to do nothing...for 20 minutes. Despite feeling exhausted and craving even a moment to sit still and rest, just thinking about doing nothing brought up fear, anxiety and agitation about what might happen.

My Storyteller fired off a bunch of thoughts starting with "I can't just do nothing because..." and "If I do that, then..." as well as "Who will do xyz while I'm just sitting and doing nothing?" It should be noted that my son was in therapy or at school for a few hours, yet these thoughts appeared even when I had time to myself and nothing that really needed to be done.

I couldn't express this back then, but what I now know is that I feared what stillness might bring up. I was scared of feeling things I had been suppressing for years. I thought that it would be too much and that I'd get "stuck in the muck of suck" around what I thought my life was turning out to be. There were also the BIG stories I was constantly creating around the lack of possibility and hope for my son's future.

I thought all of these things AND because I really wanted to feel joy again and had committed on some level to trusting in the unknown, I did it. I took my judgment of how this was a big waste of time along with all of my thoughts and fears and one Saturday morning, I passed the parental baton to my husband. I grabbed my blanket, went outside, set my timer for 20 minutes and sat in the awkward stillness. It was in the book, therefore, the rule follower in me had to do it.

My mind went crazy with all sorts of stories about what I "should" be doing instead of sitting. My Battle Ready Bodyguard created discomfort because my Storyteller was loud and convincing. It was a serious challenge not to get up and start cleaning up dog poop. Yes, you read that correctly. I had to keep myself from getting up and scooping dog poop because that was preferable to the foreign feeling of sitting and doing nothing!

Of course Martha Beck knew this would happen, so she advised the reader to just notice all of this, but not really pay attention to what the thinking mind was saying. To get out of the thinking mind and back into the body, notice the thoughts and take a deep breath. Tune into the senses. Doing this gives your brain a task to perform; it can't smell something AND worry about the future at the same time. From there, it is simply a "rinse and repeat" process.

Doing as I was told, I sat and simply noticed the thoughts that were streaming through my monkey mind. They were fascinating! There were comical thoughts along the same line as cleaning dog poop. Some were reminders of things that I had been wanting or needing to do. It was a challenge not to act on these as well and over the years, I have found a helpful strategy for this that I'll share at the end of this section.

Other thoughts struck a nerve because they were thoughts about me, my son, the past, the present, the future. I didn't know what to do with them at that point, but I now know that being aware of your Storyteller and the stories it creates, is a really important place to begin.

Why Is Stillness So Important?

Stillness creates awareness. If you can become an observer of your thoughts, of what is going on in your body as well as the reality of the present moment, you can begin to question things. You can begin to tune into what feels true and right for you (and your family) based on what is happening right here, right now.

So often we go through life either reliving the past or preparing for the future. Becoming aware of where your thoughts are and utilizing your senses to get back into your body allows you to be in the present...which happens to be the only moment you can do anything about!

Playing with this in small increments will make it easier to implement the ability to notice thoughts and get back into the present when in the midst of chaos, stress, meltdowns and other challenging times.

Are you ready to give it a try? If so, yay!! If not, it is there for you when you are ready.

I invite you to start small. Sit and do nothing for a few minutes. Find somewhere comfortable, even if this means reclining the driver's seat of your car as you wait in the carpool line. I've had times where my "nothing time" happened in the bathroom because it was the only place I could go to lock the door and be alone.

Put your phone down. Get your body comfortable and just breathe. In and out. Just sit, breathe and notice. Notice the thoughts. Notice how your body feels.

Don't do anything with your thoughts or feelings right now. You can utilize the strategies shared earlier after your stillness session. Don't pay attention to them beyond simply noticing they are there and returning to your body and senses. You don't have to do anything but sit and breathe.

The practice of stillness might require setting boundaries with the people in your life. I had to be very specific and direct with my husband that while I was sitting and doing my "nothingness," he needed to watch our son and that for the short amount of time that I was sitting, I didn't want to be disturbed. He quickly realized that this practice made me calmer, happier and better able to handle things, which was a welcome change from his perspective.

Another useful practice is known as Sit Spot, which is simply sitting outside and noticing. When my husband was not home I would sit my son near a window so he could see me outside sitting and feel safe. I also gave him a timer so he knew how long it was going to be.

There were times when he was too anxious to be alone inside so I brought him out with me. I was explicit and told him it was a quiet, sitting time for me. While I didn't want to do this all of the time, it was a wonderful opportunity for me to play with giving myself what I wanted and needed without neglecting myself because of his wants and needs. That alone was a big time meditative practice!

Play around with what works best for you and your family, gently stretching your family so that you can have a small amount of time to yourself without doing anything. It's also a modeling opportunity for them to see that it's okay to simply sit in stillness and that it can be an important part of a parent taking care of themself.

Practicing stillness might shine a light on the fact that it is more challenging for you than it is for your family members. Can you allow yourself this time? Can you ask for what you want and need?

This exercise of doing nothing can bring to the surface all sorts of thoughts and stories about what you can or cannot do. Awesome!! Tuck them away as these are juicy thoughts you'll want to revisit and question. Go do nothing anyways. You have my permission.

> If your mind is causing strong resistance to this, try a strategy I've used many times. Take a pad of paper and pencil with you, set it on your lap, don't look at it or focus on it but when anything comes to mind, jot it down without looking.
>
> You may notice your mind becomes like microwave popcorn. Nothing much happens for the first few seconds and then lots of thoughts and reminders pop up like crazy before finally slowing down.

Once you are done with your stillness session, you've got a list of all that your mind was trying to share with you. Some things might be helpful, others comical. You don't have to do anything with any of this right now. It's all just good to know and you've gotten it out of your thinking mind and on your pad of paper!

If you want to learn more about what was shared in this section on stillness, check out...

"The Joy Diet" Dr. Martha Beck,

"There's Not Enough Time...and Other Lies We Tell Ourselves" Jill Farmer

If you also always have too much to do, my dear friend and fellow master life coach, Jill Farmer, wrote this wonderful book. Check it out!!

"Sit Spot and the Art of Inner Tracking" Michael Trotta

If you are curious about my Sit Spot practice, check out this book that provides 30 days of prompts that will put your Storyteller to work in noticing things from a completely different perspective.

The Boomerang Effect of Too Much Action

In 2012 during my nature based coach training, I was introduced to a system based on natural energy cycles as described in Ellen Haas, Evan McGown and Jon Young's "Coyote's Guide to Connecting with Nature." Their system is similar to how I had learned to create and teach units and lessons way back when I studied Education at the University of Dayton and used it to plan coaching workshops, retreats and classes for my clients.

I was noticing its value with everything I did and as I played with it more and more on a daily basis, I came to realize just how important using the natural energy cycle is in parenting. I also became aware of what I refer to as the "boomerang effect" and its role in leaving me feeling exhausted and stuck.

This natural energy flow system involves looking at things in a cyclical fashion, utilizing the image of a compass rose, with each direction assigned a specific energy so that things flow naturally.

This also weaves together the energies of the four archetypes I focus on and how to use them to make the most of the energy you are putting into whatever you are doing.

- Monarch/Elder - North
- Child - East
- Warrior - South
- Teacher/Community Builder - West

Here are the directions and their associated energies:

NE - Intention Setting

E - Inspiration (the What and/or Why behind the intention)

SE - Preparation

S - Action

SW - Relaxation and Recovery

W - Celebration

NW - Reflection

N - Integration

These energies used as a complete cycle can create a flow and balance in life that feels good and also aid in truly learning and growing from our experiences.

What I noticed was that I was exhausting myself because I was "boomerang-ing" and focused on the "doing" energies of the cycle (Intention setting, Inspiration, Preparation and Action) and spending very little time in the "being" energies (Relaxation, Celebration, Reflection and Integration).

This would frequently happen when I'd hear an idea from another parent, try it out and spend a few seconds recovering from the energy spent before another suggestion or recommendation would come my way about how to better help my son. I would then boomerang right back into action mode preparing to act on the new intention I was inspired to have.

It felt extremely uncomfortable to not act on these things because everything felt so urgent with regards to supporting my son in catching up with his chronological peers. This was happening all of the time and I began to notice this with my clients as well.

> There is no such thing as catching up since brains cannot be forced to do things they are not ready for. They develop when they are ready.

I wasn't spending any time truly recovering and giving myself the care that I desperately needed, essentially time and space, even if only for a few moments. I wasn't celebrating any wins or gains or even acknowledging the fact that I was willing to try something different even if it didn't give me the result I was hoping for. I wasn't taking time to reflect on what happened in order to notice what worked, what didn't work and/or what I could do differently the next time.

Because none of these were happening, I wasn't integrating what I was learning about myself, my child, our relationship, etc. and therefore couldn't use that feedback to support us all the next time. I was constantly starting from scratch or reinventing the wheel which was not only exhausting, but it also led me to judge myself for not being able to figure anything out.

Learning how to balance the "doing" and the "being" energies can help you to feel more clarity around where your energy and attention are going while also giving yourself the time and space (even in small doses) to rest, celebrate, reflect and integrate the things that can help to make life a bit easier.

If you want to learn more about this, check out "Coyote's Guide to Connecting with Nature" by Ellen Haas, Evan McGown and Jon Young.

Part Three Conclusion: Summary, Key Concepts and Power Questions

Summary:

I hope that by getting to know when the Storyteller, the Battle Ready Bodyguard, and the Guardian of Your Heart become Shadow Forces, you have a better sense of what to do when their misguided protection keeps you stuck in thoughts, tension and feelings that aren't supporting you in being the parent you want to be.

Rather than believing painful thoughts about your situation, get curious about what your situation is trying to help you to learn or practice.

Rather than carrying tension around in your body or repressing emotions that you are feeling when annoyed or frustrated, recognize what your body is telling you and find healthy ways to release, express or create what it is that you are wanting or needing.

Awareness of how these archetypes appear in your life can help to empower you to shift them from being shadowy characters to ones that are focused on using their superpowers in ways that will create positive changes in your life. Doing this helped me tremendously and it is my hope that it will do the same for you.

Key Concepts:

- The Storyteller - Notice Thoughts that Include *Should, Need/s To, Have/Has To, Must*
- Re-Living Situations and Conversations
- Pre-Living and Future-Tripping Thoughts
- Awareness of Thoughts in the Present Moment
- Byron Katie's Inquiry Process - The Work
- Notice and Question
- Thoughts Create Physical Responses
- Body Scan - Learning Your Body's Responses to Negative and Positive Thoughts
- Using the Senses to Get Out of Your Head and Back Into the Present Moment
- The Guardian of Your Heart and Emotional Lockdown
- Margaret-ism: Pinballing
- Undercurrent of Energy
- Processing Emotions in Healthy Ways
- Importance of Stillness

Power Questions:

- Byron Katie's "The Work" - Is it true? Can I absolutely know it is true? What happens when I believe the thought? Who would I be without the thought?

- What am I making this mean?
- Is there any tension in my body? If so, where is it and what does it feel like?
- What is actually going on at this moment?
- Where are my thoughts?
- What am I trying to protect myself from or prepare myself for?
- What did that experience/situation teach me?
- What can I do to help my future self out?
- What do I know about my child that I can play with next time?
- Am I noticing and allowing myself to feel contentment, peace, ease and joy?
- What is causing me tension and what is my intention?
- What is it that I am feeling? How is this emotion trying to help or support me?

PART FOUR

Control and Judgment

In the previous part you got to know a bit more about your ever creative Storyteller, your Battle Ready Bodyguard, and the Guardian of your Heart. These characters have helped you to begin noticing your thoughts, recognize what is going on in your body and start to build a new relationship with your emotions. The tools shared to help with these all are essential to have in your parenting toolbox (or backpack) as you embark on your own hero's journey in parenting the child you did not expect while you were expecting.

Even if you have mastered these tools, you will still encounter stumbling blocks along the way. I refer to these stumbling blocks as "Hindering Forces." They are things that can trip you up and hold you back from feeling confidence and clarity under the guise of keeping you safe. This is just more of the Warrior's misguided protective care showing up.

I have found that the two biggest Hindering Forces for us as parents are control and judgment, and oh how persistent they can be! But don't worry! My intention in this section is to introduce you to the tools and strategies that, used along with what you've already learned, will help you recognize them for what they are so that you can hold onto that confidence and clarity, even in the midst of the most chaotic and challenging times when the Hindering Forces try relentlessly to convince you that they should be listened to.

Believing the Hindering Forces might cause you to question yourself.

They might send you into the "muck of suck."

They might make you feel like nothing you are doing is making a difference.

> I am here to tell you that as much as they want to protect you, they are wrong and there are other, more empowering, ways to view the challenges faced as parents.

Parenting Feels Like Kayaking…but I Don't Know How to Kayak

Since I love metaphors, here is one that always comes to mind when I think about getting stuck in a Hindering Force.

Early on in my journey, when everything felt incredibly tough and I didn't know what to do, I did what I always did. I worked really hard because that is what I thought I should do. I grew up in the midwest and it was considered to be an admirable quality to work hard and be busy.

Well, one day I realized that parenting felt like going down rapids in a kayak, something I don't know how to do, which is why everything felt so out of control and extremely hard! There were times when I tried paddling back to calmer waters and this took a ton of energy. It didn't work to help me feel better because even if I got to calmer waters, as soon as I stopped to take a breath, there I was again, swept back in, bouncing around in a current of frustration and helplessness.

There were times when I would come upon obstacles (this could be anything from realizing my son was not playing with his peers, frustrated that he wasn't yet speaking or watching the reactions of other parents to his behavior when he was anxious or excited) and get stuck.

Rather than using my paddle to steer around them, I would get out and try to manage my kayak while also trying to remove the obstacle from my path. This looked like trying harder to get him to talk and interact with his peers or not have meltdowns so I could control our experience. This was exhausting and only added to my feelings of awkwardness and incapability.

Once I connected this metaphor with parenting, not only did it seem comical, I also knew things had to change. I realized that a lot of the paddling upstream was me wanting to go back to the known. I wanted to go back to times where things felt easier, times when my son was younger and we were unaware that he was on his own developmental timeline, sitting in his stroller, with nobody else to compare our lives to.

I realized that a major obstacle to having more ease, peace and joy in my life was the constant effort I was putting into changing his developmental differences. This was an intense energy that is not at all the same as doing what I could to support his developmental differences. Based on what I was hearing and interpreting from the experts, I believed that if those differences weren't there, if he could do everything his chronological peers could do, he would be happy and have the potential to be successful in life and then I could relax and feel happy.

I had to learn to acknowledge that these differences were part of him and that a majority of the time, he was happy. He loved what he loved without apology, like looking at ceiling fans and outdoor light sconces. He did things in his own way, in his own time, and by supporting this, he was allowed to develop at a pace that supported (and continues to support) his happiness. Again, he was usually happy and content and

I was the one who needed to do things differently if I wanted to feel those things.

The kayak metaphor has helped me to be able to check in and get curious with myself when I felt that familiar tension of exhaustion and frustration. When I felt things were tense or difficult, I began to ask myself - Am I trying to paddle upstream again? Am I trying to manage my kayak while attempting to move obstacles?

If any of this was true, good to know because now I had information to help me zoom out and check in with (and question) my thoughts. I had learned how to create space between me and the obstacles and I could now pause to take some deep breaths. Doing so helped me gain greater clarity around what actually mattered to me and this helped me to relinquish the illusion of control and flow with greater ease with whatever it was that was happening.

I will be honest and say that while I am so happy to have realized this, at the time, allowing things to flow like this felt weird. There was some grieving involved around the expectations I had for what I thought parenting was going to be like and once I allowed the grief without judgment, things felt so much different. I could enjoy him exactly as he was. I could support him exactly where he was. I wasn't spending so much energy fighting, which meant I had energy to enjoy the simple and real things in our life.

Chapter Twelve

Control

As you continue wandering with greater awareness of your Warrior and the many ways it shows up, you will begin to feel more empowered as you keep your Shadow Forces at bay.

But there will be other times when you may feel like as you take any step forward, something is trying to hold you back. You will turn around to check out exactly what is causing this resistance, but see nothing except your own shadow.

You start to move again but it's as though the resistance is trying to send you a message.

Stop!
Go back!
You are going to lose control!

You really want to trust in this process so you try cautiously exploring the next step and there it is again.

Don't do it!

It's not safe!

Everything is going to fall apart!

Have you experienced this? I certainly have, especially as I started to get more curious and question the old thoughts and patterns created by my Shadow Forces. I discovered that my Warrior was at it again, this time as a Hindering Force, attempting to keep me safe by trying to maintain some illusion of control. While the intention comes from a well-meaning place, it creates a lot of unnecessary tension.

When you are parenting a child whose developmental timeline, personality or learning styles are unique OR parenting is simply not what you expected while you were expecting, things tend to feel chaotic and out of control. This feels uncomfortable, so you grasp at anything that you feel is under your control.

At first, this reactive place is a survival mechanism in order to be able to get through the day and all of the challenges faced with parenting. If something worked and you had some sort of influence over it, you store it in your memory vault as "necessary for survival."

> Utilizing what worked as feedback is very different from making them universal laws that must be obeyed at all times.

If you are not aware of your intention and true motivation—your reason for doing the things that ended up working —you can slide down the slippery slope of becoming a control freak...like I was!

As I have shared, when my own journey in parenting began, very little was going as described in any of the parenting books or checklists that I had access to. I felt like I was literally playing a never-ending game of Whack-A-Mole, reacting to whatever popped up and making everything up on the fly. If something worked and a metaphorical mole got whacked, whatever I had done became THE way of doing it, even if it was just a coincidence. Dirty looks were administered if anyone questioned or strayed from the way I did things.

> As you wander through this journey, you will most likely experience others on their journey feeling just as uncertain. They may share what has worked for them in order to get confirmation that they have made the right choices for their children. This can create confusion or doubt that you are parenting your child in the right way. Every child is so different and each of our journeys are meant to teach us what we need. To this, I say, stay open, curious, aware and connected to your intention and what feels true in your gut.

Looking back, I spent a lot of unproductive Warrior energy trying to control things. This is where knowing about the Shadow Forces (the Storyteller, Battle Ready Bodyguard and the Guardian of Your Heart) is helpful because the Hindering

Forces love to employ them to support their mission to keep you safe.

My Storyteller would create stories about what "might" happen, so I would plan obsessively in order to try and prepare myself.

My Battle Ready Bodyguard would get involved and have me pre-experience anxiety around things that hadn't happened yet, things that may never happen.

The Guardian of my Heart did what it could, often counting on the other forces to protect me from feeling sad, disappointed and embarrassed.

Sound familiar? If so, you are not alone! Just for fun, take a second and just allow your mind to think about all of the things that you try to control or believe you have control over.

These are things I personally did to try and control situations:

- We would get to school at a certain time so that my child was the first to be on the swing because it helped him to regulate his body before school. This helped me believe that he would do great while in school. I also believed that if he wasn't able to do this, his day would get off to a bad start and I would get texts throughout the day from teachers.
- I felt like I was the only one who could do anything for my child, even though I had a husband and a support system who were wonderful, because I

thought they wouldn't do it right and I would have to deal with the aftermath.

- I felt a great deal of anxiety and apprehension around going out for an evening or a vacation with my husband or a friend because I felt nobody else could possibly care for my child. He had apraxia of speech and didn't speak consonants until 5 so I worried they wouldn't know what he wanted...despite the fact that he was better at conveying his wants than I was!

- I organized and decluttered my house like crazy because it was the only thing I could do to feel in control of at least one aspect of my life. The Container Store was my favorite place to go back then because there were so many things that helped me feel like I could simplify life and contain things that felt chaotic.

The reality of life is that you actually don't control anything other than your thoughts and reactions. You have complete control of whether or not to believe your Storyteller's creations about what is going on around you, so with that knowledge, questioning those stories becomes important.

You also have control over the actions you do or do not take. You might feel like you can or have been able to control things; however, as much as I would love to congratulate you on being the first person to do so, you cannot control everything! You can do what you can to lead a situation or influence an outcome, but that is very different from control.

> My favorite reframe on this is, "What can I do to influence this situation or experience?" This conveys much different energy and is more effective than trying to control.

You also might have created stories of other parents who appear to have control of their kids. They do not. Their kids might be people pleasers, rule followers, fearful or just have a different personality that may be more easy going. If the parent controls through fear or threats, they may feel successful when the child is a child, however, the trauma of that will not be helpful in supporting the child in growing into a well adjusted adult.

Let's think about what happens in your body when you are trying to control something. Does it feel loose, relaxed, open and expansive to possibility or does your Battle Ready Bodyguard take over and cause it to feel tight and constricted with narrow vision, no curiosity or openness and shallow breath? The latter is what I felt so often and just like with the kayak metaphor, it kept me from noticing what I could do that would actually be helpful and using my time, energy and attention more effectively and efficiently.

There were many times when I was using these things - my time, energy and attention - in ways to control my interactions with other people. This gave me what I call "Shadow Payoffs" which are things I was wanting or needing (time, space, compassion) but going about getting them in a shadowy manner because I wasn't allowing myself to admit that I wanted or needed things or I simply just didn't know. I'm not proud of these patterns that emerged but also know I'm not alone.

Margaret-ism
Shadow Payoffs

As you continue along your journey you may notice things about yourself or become aware of patterns of how you go about things that don't feel great. You may see yourself…

- worrying more about what other people think than using what you know about your child

- getting defensive with others in your life who simply ask a question

- being snarky with your partner or child when they ask you to do something

- feeling like a martyr and gathering evidence of all that you do that goes unnoticed, underappreciated and doesn't make a difference anyway

Personally, I played the role of a martyr quite well with a consistent undercurrent of energy in the form of "overwhelm." I did this in order to control and keep everyone's expectations low. Why? Because if I was overwhelmed, then most likely no one would expect x, y or z of me.

Sure there were times when I genuinely felt overwhelmed but more often than not, my Storyteller was hard at work re-living and pre-living situations during conversations with family members in order to get attention and sympathy.

If doing this sounds and feels at all familiar to you it's because it is a commonly used defensive strategy. It is just your Warrior trying to be helpful...yet again.

When I notice this in myself, my favorite question to ask is...

What is the shadow payoff for doing this or being this way?

It may surprise you, as it did me, to discover that I was doing lots of things that didn't feel so great because of the shadow payoffs I was getting. These are just unhealthy patterns that can be turned around once recognized for what they are.

When I began paying more attention to how I was showing up throughout the day in my life, I noticed that there were times I was being snarky with my husband and son, putting out an undercurrent of energy of annoyance and frustration. What would happen as a result of this? Well, my husband would pick up on this, leave me alone and take over with our son.

So what was actually going on? When I zoomed out, I realized that I was wanting, or rather needing, a time-out, time to myself because I was feeling overwhelmed, tired, annoyed or just done. Rather than just asking for a few minutes of quiet, alone time to regroup, I was behaving in a way that got me to a place where people were leaving me alone (the shadow payoff), however, it was achieved in a way that felt crappy to all involved.

While this was humbling to realize that there was some form of unconscious manipulation happening on my part, it was also quite freeing for me. When I recognized certain shadow behaviors emerging, I could do something different, something less manipulative, in order to try and get what I was actually needing and/or wanting.

When you can ask in clear and specific ways for what you need, without the undercurrent of energy being snark or irritation, it feels so much better! Even if it is not possible at the moment, you now know what you need and can get curious about how to give it to yourself sometime soon...even if it is five minutes alone in the bathroom.

> We aren't the only ones who get shadow payoffs for things, our children do as well. I will share more about that later but for now, it's helpful to have on your radar when your child does something and you are left wondering why on earth they would have done it. Perhaps there was a shadow payoff involved in the form of attention (positive or negative), engagement, reaction, etc.

We are now going to explore some tools that you can use when the Hindering Force of Control takes over.

Tool #1: TIANT Process

I first heard the phrase "Intention. Attention. No Tension at the Equus retreat I described earlier. Popularized by the prolific self-help author Marci Shimoff, the phrase is used most often in Transformational Coaching to help people be more effective in achieving their goals---greater clarity in exactly what it is you want to achieve (Intention) leads to a perspective shift (Attention) that helps focus on the means to achieve your goal, while letting go of the expectations, concerns, negativities, etc. that get in the way of achieving that goal (No Tension).

I realized that the concepts in the phrase could be expanded to fit my own understanding by first acknowledging the role tension plays in the process of setting intentions and directing attention and awareness. This is especially important in parenting because I can have an intention, give it all of the attention I want but still not get any closer to what I am wanting for myself, my child or my family because I haven't addressed what is causing tension or creating a disconnect between reality and intention in the first place.

I have found it to be empowering to start with identifying the tension because doing so allows me to connect reality with intention in order to create more doable and realistic ways to focus my attention while not having a tight grasp on the outcome...no (or less) tension. Acknowledging that something is not working and causing me tension is powerful because it is only from the place of recognizing this that I can choose to do something different.

Conscious noticing of this shakes me out of the fog of stories and beliefs that my Storyteller has created and from there I can check in with my intention and ask the power question I shared before for this...

- *What is it that I'm/we're actually wanting?*

Once I have gotten clarity around what I am actually wanting, I can start to get curious about what I can influence in this particular situation. I can ask...

- *Where can I place my attention that would be helpful in supporting my intention?*
- *What attention can I give to this?*
- *What specifically does this look like or require based on the reality of the present moment or circumstances?"*

After that, I can allow myself to experience no (or less) tension by releasing any expectations I may have or needs I have for things to go or be a certain way in order for me to flow with what is happening. I can learn from the feedback that I'm getting and try something else. This is where tremendous learning can take place.

Doing this allows me to have more peace, ease and joy, regardless of what is going on. I have been utilizing what I now call the TIANT Process and it helps me each and every day in every aspect of my life, especially parenting.

The TIANT Process stands for...

Tension - What is something that is causing tension in your life?

Intention - What are you wanting to feel or experience? Where are you trying to go? What is the goal? (Please be as realistic as possible knowing yourself, your child, your family, etc.)

Attention - What are all of the things that you can realistically do to support your intention? Doing this considering everyone involved can be very helpful!

No (or less) Tension - Release the need for things to go as expected in order to flow with reality.

Personal Parenting Example of Using the TIANT Process:

Tension

What is something that is causing tension in your life?

My son often forgets to charge his electronics which leads to meltdowns if they aren't working when he wants to use them, which leads to a lot of tension for me, especially when I am trying to get something done or on a client call.

Intention

What are you wanting to feel or experience? Where are you trying to go? What is the goal? (Please be as realistic as possible knowing yourself, your child, your family, etc.)

I am wanting us all to feel prepared and able to do what we are wanting and needing to do. Why do I want this? It will feel so much better for everyone!

Attention

What are all of the things that you can realistically do to support your intention? Doing this considering everyone involved can be very helpful!

- *Create a central hub for electronics to charge.*
- *Create reminders and alarms for him to remind him to charge his things before bedtime.*
- *Make sure there are chargers in the spaces that these electronics go.*
- *Charge things overnight so they are ready for the next day.*

No (or Less) Tension

Release the need for things to go as expected in order to flow more with reality.

- *Acknowledge that I cannot control whether or not he listens to the reminders or alarms or actually plugs them in to charge and do my best to stay calm and not get tangled up in his strong emotions when something dies.*
- *I can also get perspective when a device does die that pressing pause on what I'm doing is not the end of the world. Maybe my client will understand, maybe even appreciate me more as a trusted resource because I understand what they go through with their own child when they see I need to pause a session to help him.*

This is how I approach my life, whether it's related to my son, my family, my home, my business, my travels, our holidays, etc. Thinking about something that causes me tension allows me to be more intentional and also be more proactive about where to place my attention as opposed to "pinballing" around like I used to.

When I try to control things, I am out of the present moment and am in no position to be agile and curious about what is possible. When I press pause and think about what is actually causing me tension, I can get more clear about my intention and curious about what I have influence over and then things change almost immediately. I feel much more flexible and empowered.

Sometimes crazy stuff gets thrown my way and it might not be super fun. Being able to employ my Monarch/Elder and Child archetypes allows me to have access to a big picture perspective and curiosity around possibilities for solutions. This is a powerful thing to model for my child because he can learn by watching my own reactions and understand that even adults, his parents, cannot control anything but our thoughts and the actions we take.

The ability to let go of any ideas that we might have around controlling others or circumstances in our lives is freeing. It actually allows us to be more effective and efficient with what we do, with whatever comes up. Who doesn't want that?

Tool #2: Relinquishing Control and Building Your Support Network

The inability to relinquish control is a common source of tension for the parents I work with in my coaching practice. Many with children who are on their own developmental timeline have difficulty allowing others to care for their child.

The Storyteller likes to create all sorts of thoughts about how nobody else will be able to handle them. The Guardian of your Heart also gets involved and tells you that you might get hurt by allowing someone into the reality of what your life is really like. This of course activates the Bodyguard who then creates all sorts of boundaries and challenges so that this cannot happen.

I completely relate to this all as I had many stories around what would or could happen to my son if I wasn't there to watch him closely. No one else could possibly be able to understand his apraxic utterances to know that what he was asking for was apple juice in a purple cup with a pink straw.

Because of this all, I had set major boundaries. I wouldn't let anyone except close family come over because I couldn't guarantee that my son would have clothes on or that he wouldn't be having a meltdown. My Bodyguard and Guardian of my Heart teamed up and were on full alert, protecting my heart and ego from feeling any sort of discomfort or defensiveness around who and how he was, as well as my parenting of him.

This changed once I began to notice and question the thoughts and stories of my Storyteller. With practice, I started allowing others to support us. I began to relieve my Bodyguard of its duty, loosening the reins a bit as I gathered evidence of how my son was okay when I wasn't around to meet all of his needs and wants. Turns out, there was quite a bit of evidence that he could find ways to get exactly what he wanted or needed without words better than I could with them.

When I did not allow others to support him (and me), I was actually denying all of us opportunities to learn and grow. With others, he learned how to communicate and express himself in different ways. When I denied others from getting to be with him and learn from him, I was also denying them the chance to hang out with a kid who was really interesting and fun to be with.

Relinquishing control triggered all aspects of my Warrior big time. My Storyteller, Battle Ready Bodyguard and the Guardian of my Heart went into high protective mode, so I started with super small steps to try to keep them calm.

I invited caregivers, who were usually college aged children of people I knew and trusted, to come over and play with him.

I was still nearby, doing random things like laundry or checking email, which allowed me to ease any discomfort I had around thoughts like, *"What will happen if he is not understood? What will happen if he has a meltdown?"* I was close so that I could step in to support them if needed.

> If you are lucky enough to live in or near a college town, you might consider contacting the heads of the psychology or social work or education or occupational therapy, etc. departments to see if they are interested in alerting their students to the sort of opportunities that I was able to utilize for my son. While I was studying education I frequently babysat and tutored in order to gain experience and earn some spending money.

My nervousness quickly vanished as I realized that the people who were playing with him were fun and had far more energy than I did to do the things he wanted to do. They were also there for short amounts of time. Their job was to play with him. They weren't distracted by things like cleaning, laundry, making meals or any of the many things that would catch my attention as soon as I sat down to play with him. Since I could get a lot of those things done while they were at our house, when they left, I was able to give him more of my energy and attention.

These caregivers became part of our family and he loved being with them all. While most of the time was spent having fun, they all experienced challenging times with him. Almost all of them were interested in education, occupational therapy, speech pathology or social work.

They were helping me out and I like to think that we were also helping them out. They got to experience the reality of caring for a child who was on his own developmental timeline. They also got to experience a child who probably didn't respond in the same way that other children did. They learned that he could not be controlled and wasn't easily distracted or going to forget once he set his mind on something. With my support, they figured out plans for what to do the next time so everyone was on the same page and ready for any challenges that might arise.

I remember many situations around filming ceiling fans at a nearby hotel attached to our neighborhood club. He was adamant on the order he would see them and if he ran out of room on his phone, would expect to start all over again. If this was not possible, strong emotional reactions ensued. The sitters all learned how to handle these meltdowns beautifully, while also acknowledging how tough it was in the moment. This confirmed for me that I wasn't the only one who struggled at times with my son.

My initial worries and fears had us living in the shadow energy of the Teacher/Community Builder archetype and if I had listened to my Storyteller, I would have kept us both from expanding our network of supportive people. He wouldn't have gotten to have all of the fun experiences he had or learn from different people who approached things in different ways.

Relinquishing my own desire to control and the thought that I was the only one who could take care of him, was a huge weight lifted off of my back. As a result, I had more energy and time for myself. In addition to that, my son has learned how to be more flexible and to feel safe and cared for even when I am not there. How is that for a turnaround?!?!

Tool #3: Creating Flow Through Awareness of Needs (Parent and Child)

I can recall a trip I took alone with my son to visit my sister. We travel together frequently and on this particular trip, I began to notice an undercurrent of tension-filled energy for me. When I got curious, it consisted of anxiety, frustration and annoyance around preparing his backpack.

Why? It never failed that as soon as we got 15 minutes from our house or into the airport and through security, he would ask if I had packed specific things for him. If I hadn't, he would have a meltdown. This of course brought up more anxiety for me and lots of storytelling around getting kicked off the plane and never being able to travel with him again. It was the same scenario every single time!

After listening to a TiLT Parenting podcast with Deborah Reber and Seth Perler on the topic of executive functioning, which is basically the ability to plan, organize, remember steps and follow through to get things done, I realized a few things. While I couldn't change the challenges my son had with planning or his anxiety around not having his stuff, there were things I could do differently.

I took a few minutes to go through the TIANT Process in order to see what I could do differently. Reflecting on the things that typically created tension —which were usually the same each time— I was then able to utilize my own executive functioning strategies in order to support us both.

Getting curious about his needs and wants helped me shift things. Instead of me taking on the responsibility of packing for him, I began to make this something he was part of so that he had a tangible experience in the process. I created a list of tasks geared towards helping him to get prepared for the trip. These were specific, appropriate and doable for him, which is important to keep in mind regardless of chronological age.

Here are some examples of things he could gather or take care of ahead of time:

- Putting snacks in his lunchbox along with an empty cup and straw;
- Getting the electronics he wanted to bring ready by making sure there was enough storage and that he had the right chargers (including portable chargers) and cords for them;
- Thinking about the entertainment he wanted for the plane ride so we could download movies and bring headphones;
- Gathering small toys (like tops) or stuffed animals, coloring books or activity book with crayons or markers;

I would begin this process a week before (if possible) so that I didn't feel stressed or rushed and because I've learned that to help my future self out, there were a couple of different phases involved in this packing preparation.

Example:

- If he wanted special snacks on the plane, I needed time to get them from the store.

- We needed to update his iPad days before, not the night before because this takes time and an internet connection.

- We made sure there was room on his iPad so that we could download movies or shows to watch, like his favorite shows from the HGTVGo app, "Property Brothers" or "Love It or List It."

Of course there were always some minor things that popped up, like not knowing where his shoes were as we were trying to get out of the door.

Taking time to think about what was going on during these "Groundhog's Day-like" scenarios changed my approach to this whole process and removed a great deal of pressure from me. This meant that I could relax a bit and not feel that tension-filled undercurrent of energy with him as we walked into the airport. He knew exactly what was in his backpack and what was available for him to eat, do and watch.

Now when we travel, he makes his own packing list of what he needs a week or two before a trip and together, we make sure things get done as best as we can!

Chapter Thirteen

Judgment

Most of the Hero's Journey can leave you feeling like you are all alone because, unless you are fortunate enough to have a connection with other parents who "get it", you are usually surrounded by parents who are more or less oblivious to the challenges you are encountering. Their parenting experience involves activities where they can sit together, chat and watch their children play, while we are usually on high alert for our child's meltdowns, strong emotional reactions, stress-inducing transitions from one thing to another, or the isolating effects of not being able to participate because of a developmental difference.

In addition to this loneliness, it can also be as if you are living in a fishbowl. You may feel as though everyone is watching you, judging you for what you are doing or not doing as a parent. This can create traces of self doubt, even after you've taken steps forward to help yourself and your child. Don't get me wrong, every parent has their worries, but when parenting children like ours, these worries tend to be magnified and tend to attract unwanted attention.

Judgment is something that we all do and is part of human nature. We have to judge distances and time. We have to judge whether or not something is good to ingest. We have to judge whether or not someone is trustworthy. Judgment helps us to be aware of things that could harm us.

Judgment can come from one's own internal rules. As I shared earlier, these are things taught directly or indirectly to us or other people around us about how something or someone "should" be, what they "should" behave like or what they "should" do.

> These internal rules can also be the creations of our Storyteller so it's important to recognize that judgment comes from a thought, a person's perspective or from their past experiences AND it is not the same as fact.

A common example of this is someone telling you that your child "should" be able to just eat what is put in front of them. "They "should" just eat it and if they refuse, they shouldn't eat at all. They'll figure it out when they get hungry. Simple."

Or noticing judgmental internal thoughts about your parenting or your child while at a gathering with friends, "Their children eat whatever is on their plate. What am I doing wrong!? Why can't my child just eat what is offered? Why do they have to be so difficult?"

I cannot tell you how many times I have heard these statements and felt the judgment of others around this one issue. My son, like many neurodiverse individuals, has sensory challenges around food.

These statements and thoughts may work fine if you have a child who does not have sensory or other challenges around food, but when your child struggles with these things, it isn't "simple." Many children with sensory issues are simply incapable of overcoming the sensory overload issues that make certain foods aversive to them such as food that feels, smells or tastes gross, icky, too strong, different, etc. to them. (These are all descriptions my son has given to food we have presented him with over the years.) As parents, we can then find ourselves in a situation where our child isn't getting the nutrition and calories that they need to grow.

The good thing is, there are ways to approach food in order to support the child. Forcing or shaming them to eat food their body and brain is not ready for - whatever the reason - is not the way to do this, regardless of what you or others think.

> We did a "food school" with his OT, based on Dr. Kay Toomey's "SOS Approach to Feeding," and it allowed the children to essentially go back to playing with food in order to get to know it with as many senses as possible so they could feel less anxiety around what will happen when a certain food enters their mouth. While we didn't follow all of the rules of this program, we did incorporate a lot of things that allowed our son to expand his food repertoire.

Regardless of where the judgment is directed, when people judge, it usually comes from lack of knowledge, understanding and awareness. It comes from a desire to control something that feels unexpected or threatening in some way. We fear what we don't understand and we try to find comfort or understanding by trying to control the unknown which often comes through as judgments.

Realizing that this is what is actually going on when judgmental comments or looks come your way can support you in choosing to give your time and energy to yourself, your child and your family...not the judgmental person.

Navigating the Perfect Storm of Judgment in Parenting

As parents and caregivers, there are many things we experience on a day to day basis that can cause judgment and self doubt. If there is an internal rule and that rule is not followed, it can create what I call a judgment storm in parenting. This storm is when...

- You feel judged by those around you.
- You feel your child is being judged by those around you.
- You judge yourself.
- You judge your child.

Example:

It was 2006 and we were in Phoenix for my husband's neurosurgical spine fellowship and our son was almost three years old. There was a party thrown by one of the attending physicians and not being somebody who loves things like this, I quickly found my friend who was chatting with a group of ladies.

One woman was talking about potty training and how getting a child to potty train by a certain age was no big deal. Well, it sure wasn't happening for us regardless of Cheerios thrown in the toilet, potty seats around our apartment or DVD players in the bathroom. I said, "Potty training, shmotty training" and quickly learned that the woman who had been speaking had just written a book on how any child could be potty trained by a certain age.

I experienced a few feelings at the same time...as I have at many times as a parent. At first I felt bad that I had said something like that in front of her...but it was truly what I was thinking.

I felt judged by those who were in that group because they all had children who they had clearly been able to potty train---and I clearly hadn't been capable of potty training mine!

I judged myself as a mom for not being able to figure this all out. I wasn't trying hard enough or being on top of things enough.

I judged my son for not being able to do this like other children his age.

(What is so ironic about this all is that potty training is a brain development thing and I was at a party with a bunch of neurosurgeons.)

Anyways, eventually I got to the point where I could laugh about it and say something like, "Well, she is more than welcome to take my child and get him potty trained but my hunch is that she would have as much success as I am having."

Fast forward a few years and he was potty trained. He did so because his brain was ready and not because it was something I could force.

The judgment storm in parenting happens! It doesn't do anything to support either me or my son AND is something I am now extremely mindful of.

Margaret-ism
Radar Tool

This is something I came up with a few years ago and find it to be so helpful in my life because it is something I bump up against all of the time - the realization that not everything that is on my radar screen is on someone else's radar and vice versa.

Imagine that your brain is a radar screen and everything that is on your to-do list, mentally and physically, would have a dot to represent it. Your radar screen is unique to you just as mine is unique to me. Some people's radar screens have a few dots, others have many dots. This is not only interesting to consider, it also can be helpful in making sense of situations and relationships that cause tension.

How so? Well, oftentimes what we feel is important or what we are giving our attention to is not the same as other people in our lives. My radar screen would contain a lot of dots as I think about my family and their wants/needs, my pets wants/needs, my clients, my business, my friends, my home, groceries to purchase, tasks to do, travels or holidays to plan and organize, etc.

My husband's or son's brain on a radar screen would most likely contain three or four very specific dots. Not only are their radar screens different from mine, what would be on my husband's screen would not be on my son's screen, AND they would both think that what was on theirs would be the most important...because they are to them!

That is the thing with our radar screens, there are all things that we notice and feel are important. I have learned over time (and many frustrating experiences) that I can assume that others know all of the things that I am taking care of, feel strongly about or are important in keeping my child safe, but since these things aren't on their radars, they don't think of them or place the same level of importance on them like I do.

Knowing this doesn't mean that I have to suck it up and do everything on my own. It just means that if I want others to help me out, I need to be specific and ask them to support me with some of the dots on my radar.

This awareness is also helpful when considering sibling and friend relationships for your children. Your child might be frustrated that someone doesn't like something as much as they do (or the other way around) and letting them know that it just might not be on their friend or sibling's radar could be a good opportunity to introduce ways they could invite someone else to be part of something they enjoy or to see that it's not something the friend or sibling (or your child if it's flipped) wants on their radar right now and that's okay too.

Play with this and see if it makes a difference to be aware of your radar screen and the radar screens of others in your life.

> This isn't just helpful with partners and children. It is helpful with extended family members, caregivers, teachers, therapists, medical professionals and staff, co-workers, etc.

This is all good to know but when you are in a judgment storm, how do you survive and get out of it? I have found that there are a few questions that always put my Storyteller's curiosity to work in ways that are far more kind and loving for me than remaining in the judgment zone.

Question #1: Byron Katie's "Whose Business Am I In?" Model

I have already shared Byron Katie's Inquiry Process and she also has other questions that really helped me to notice how unhelpful and counterproductive judgment is in my life, especially as a mom. With practice, I began to question everything and you can too!

There are two parts of what she shares that really resonate with me around this...

1. Whose business am I in?
2. What painful thought or story am I believing or telling myself?

The "business" part is all about the three kinds of business in life:

1. My business - What I have the most influence over.
2. Other people's business - What I have very little influence over.
3. God's/Universe's business - What I have basically no influence over (weather, diagnoses, death, etc.).

I like to imagine each kind of business having their own metaphorical hula hoop in order to keep it more playful while getting curious about which hoop I am in. You may drift out of your "hoop" into other people's "hoops" (which also includes our children's business) or God's/Universe's "hoop" and this results in should-ing, trying to control, over thinking and spending precious energy on things you cannot control.

Example:

While we were not invited to many birthday parties, when we were my son didn't want to play with the other kids or do the activities, unless it had bouncy things. He only wanted to wander the house looking in each room to see if they had ceiling fans or cool light fixtures. This created so much tension for me because I had an internal rule that it was rude to go wandering through someone's home, especially bedrooms. I also worried about what the parents would think of him and his wandering.

In situations like this I began to get curious about whose business I was in and it was fascinating how busy my Storyteller was creating painful thoughts or stories about this innocent and curiosity driven desire of my son.

Whose business was I in?

I was in the birthday party host's business thinking about how they must be annoyed that he is going through each of their rooms.

I was in my son's business thinking that he should not be doing that and should just stay in the main area with the other kids.

My business in this situation is doing what I can to respect the host and their home by supporting my son in learning social rules around being in other people's homes.

It is also my business to use what I know about my son's interests and do what I can to influence the situation in a positive way for all.

- *This would include preparing him in advance by being explicit and direct about what we were going to do and where we were going to be in the home.*
- *I would have a conversation with the host about his interests so that if he did start to wander, they would know that he was just looking for ceiling fans and light fixtures.*
- *I would stay with him throughout the party to be sure he was respecting the host's home and their rules.*
- *If he could not do this, I would know that it is okay to choose in advance not to attend or if*

*things went south while we were there, we
could leave early.*

The reality was that I couldn't control my son's thinking that it was the coolest thing ever to actually be allowed to go into someone else's house and see what fans and lights they had but there were things I could do knowing he was thinking this!

Staying in "my business" always feels better because it's the only business I can actually influence. I can notice my own thoughts and decide if they are helping or hurting me. I can notice the creative stories my Storyteller is crafting when I jump into other people's business by trying to figure out what they think about me.

Being in other people's business is not at all helpful and is a huge waste of resources (time, energy, attention) that could be used for yourself and your family.

Question #2: What Am I Making it Mean?

One of my favorite questions to ask myself when I start feeling judged, like by someone who keeps looking over at us when my son makes a mucus clearing sound when he is overwhelmed, is...

What am I making it mean?

This question will usually lead to a painful thought or story, usually involving the word "should" in it. What I might make it mean when people turn and look at us could include...

- I should be able to control my child and the sounds he makes.
- We should never disturb anyone else with his sounds and should just stay home.
- My child should not clear the mucus in his throat when we are in public.

Good to know!

From there, I can ask myself the basic questions that Byron Katie came up with that I shared during the "Storyteller" section...

1. Is it true? (only answer yes or no)

2. Can I know that it is absolutely true? (only answer yes or no)

3. What happens when I believe the thought or story? How do I feel in my body? How do I treat or talk to myself? How do I treat or talk to others?

4. What would life be like without that thought or story? Who would I be in this moment without it? How would I feel in my body? How would I treat or talk to myself? How would I treat or talk to my child/spouse/partner/checkout person?

Example - I should be able to control my child and the sounds he makes.

Turnaround - I should not be able to control my child and the sounds he makes.

Evidence - I cannot control another human being and what they do. I have tried it and it doesn't work! Thinking that I can control him only makes me feel inadequate and adds tension to an already annoying experience (because I am not crazy about the sounds he makes either but I also enjoy going places).

> I want to be clear that just because we cannot predict or control our children's challenging emotional displays or behaviors does not mean that we simply do nothing. I AM suggesting, however, that letting go of the notion that we are responsible for controlling when and where they occur helps alleviate the painful feelings of negative judgments we place on ourselves and the judgments we perceive coming from others. The real value of realizing that I am not in control of what my son does lies in the way it shifts my energy from a controlling energy that ramps him up, to a calmer, more supportive energy. This allows me to focus with greater clarity on trying different strategies to see how together we can learn more adaptive ways for him to express his frustrations, anxieties, fears, etc.

You are the Expert of Your Own Child

Judgment tends to bring up challenges with trusting yourself as being a leader for your children. There are experts who are specialists in their fields AND you are the expert of your child. This is when embracing the Monarch/Elder archetypal energy comes into play as you are the one who has a lifetime of information about your child - what works for them, what doesn't, what their past experiences were like, what you have tried, what their strengths are, what their challenges are, etc.

So often parents leave appointments and meetings with doctors or other experts feeling tension around not being heard. Or they may feel like their child is not understood or accepted. Oh, and there are the worries about what the professionals think about you and how you parent.

Keep in mind, however, that the negative thoughts that might pop into your head following an encounter with an expert have no validity unless you choose to "own" those thoughts, i.e. choose to believe that the expert really did have those negative judgmental thoughts (not likely) AND that the expert's judgment about you is correct (again, not likely). As you continue to embrace curiosity, the easier it is to notice your thoughts and question them. Taking control of your thoughts in this way inevitably leads to becoming more confident in yourself as a parent.

When you start, it can feel tricky because the judgments that you feel most likely trigger your greatest insecurities. These are the things that you probably worry about the most, such as a thought like, "Am I truly doing enough?" When you explore and question this, you will almost always see that you ARE doing all that you can to support your child in a realistic manner. Other people don't know your child or the full picture of your situation, so remember that.

My goal is always to know what feels true for me, my son, our family and our life. It becomes much easier to not give a s#!t about what other people think when I am clear on those things. In order to get there, I had to learn to question a lot of my own thoughts and stories and filter out other people's judgments.

You also have within you the wisdom and the capability to filter the information that you gather from the field experts (doctors, therapists, teachers, etc.) in order to make decisions that are best for your child and your family which brings me to another powerful question.

Question #3: Am I Handing Over My Power?

If you are anything like me, when you are in the heat of challenging situations with your child, the last thing you need to be doing is giving your power away to others - family, friends, professionals, strangers, etc.

Challenging situations require every ounce of energy and attention you have to take care of yourself (through deep breaths, slowing down, etc.) so that you can take care of your child.

Unfortunately, what often happens during these times is that we tend to get distracted by (and give undue credence to) the thoughts and opinions offered by those around us. You may start worrying about what others think of you and your child. You then lose perspective and are unable to determine what is needed in the current challenging situation.

When you notice this happening, ask yourself...

- *Who am I handing my power over to?*
- *Who becomes more important than what I know?*
- *Whose opinion becomes more significant than my child?*

When my son was 7 years old, he would often start perseverating on something or have a meltdown and at that age, people began to judge more and more. Instead of calming myself so I could support him, I would worry about what friends and family members were thinking about us.

> What I have learned over the years is that they weren't judging, they often felt rather helpless and didn't know what to do to support us.

There were many times when things like this would happen out in public and strangers would actually judge us, making comments and shooting dirty looks toward me and my son. Being a recovering people pleaser, this always stung. I hated thinking we were bothering other people. However, I have realized that giving my energy and attention to people who are rude in those ways is not productive or effective and a huge waste of time.

I can't educate someone during a challenging time. I can't change how others behave. When my energy and attention is being used to tend to other people, I cannot do what I know. When I place their needs above what I know, it only makes things worse. I need to remember what I know in order to do my best to handle the situation at hand.

Realizing this changed everything for me because I was giving my energy and attention over to others, even those who didn't deserve it. Those people were usually the ones who didn't take the time to understand, consider that there might be something else going on or ask questions from a genuinely curious place. They didn't even try to empathize before inserting themselves into our challenging situation with their internal rules and expectations about how things should be handled based on their own life experiences and need to control.

During challenging times it is absolutely crucial that I NOT give my power away! What does help is bringing my energy inwards and notice that this moment is happening. It helps me to press pause and take a deep breath so that I can remember all that I know about my child and what works for him. It helps me to get clear about my intention in that moment and that is what actually makes a difference.

Handing power over can also happen in situations with experts. Below are two linked scenarios that were extremely annoying and challenging yet taught me some very important lessons as the parent of my son...

Experts Aren't *Always* Experts

When my son was around 4 years old, it was recommended by the school he attended that he get additional information about why he wasn't speaking yet. This was in the form of a neuropsychiatric evaluation and an MRI to rule out anything structurally that might be going on in his brain.

Being a rule follower, I scheduled these and they were both a complete joke. Despite explaining to the neuropsychiatrist in our pre-evaluation meeting that he did not speak, the standardized test that was administered essentially needed him to speak.

He was extremely anxious about doing anything without me in the room, so I was there, sitting and listening to the whole thing. While I could understand what he was saying, including a comment about the woman who was giving him the assessment having "triangle hair," I was not allowed to say anything or even translate what he was saying. I found this fascinating especially when she asked me to tell her what he was saying when she picked up on the fact that he was telling me something about her.

The whole thing lasted about 45 minutes and a few weeks later we received the report which basically restated everything I had filled out in the pre-evaluation paperwork. They gave him a diagnosis of PDD-NOS, Pervasive Developmental Disorder - Not Otherwise Specified, which at the time meant nothing. It also indicated that due to his inability to speak, they could not provide information on his intelligence beyond what information I had given them. I wish I had known this before spending $2500 on this. Good to know!

The next learning experience came soon after in the form of his MRI. Despite my husband being a neurosurgeon, I thought I could handle this appointment on my own, trusting the professionals to know what they were doing since they do this all of the time. I could not have been more wrong!

We arrived on time and I should have known things would not go well when the nurse taking his temperature and blood pressure got annoyed because he wouldn't sit still and that despite giving me looks as though I could do anything about this, he was not having any part of this process.

They finally got what they needed and took us back to our room where they ended up using a syringe in his mouth to give him the medicine that was supposed to make him calm and/or drowsy. Neither of these things happened as he played with some toys I had brought so they continued to give him more and more. I didn't know to question this or that I could say "No." Again, I put my trust in the people who do this every day.

Well, the MRI didn't happen and they sent me home with a drugged up child who couldn't walk but was not aware of this so as I carried him into the house and set him on the carpet, he tried crawling but his arms couldn't fully support his weight. This meant he could smack his chin on the floor if I didn't do something fast. I ran to our bedroom which was a few feet away, grabbed our pillows and created a barrier between him and the stone tile floors. I placed him as far from the tile as possible and then ran to my car in the garage to get the stroller out of the trunk and hurried back inside the house.

He had gotten to the pillow barrier but fortunately didn't get past it. I strapped him into the stroller so he would be safe and he fell asleep for about 20 minutes. While he did that, I panicked as I created a story that he might not come out of that state, that they could've damaged his brain with all of the drugs they had given him. Fortunately, that wasn't the case but it sure did wake me up to some uncomfortable realities, the main one being that the professionals don't always know best.

I told my husband what had happened and he couldn't believe that they continued to try and medicate him when it clearly wasn't working. We rescheduled the MRI to be done under proper sedation and my husband went along to make sure they didn't try talking me out of doing it another way, which they did (How messed up it that?!?!) and he said, "No. This is how it is going to happen." And that is how his

MRI was performed and showed no signs of stroke or brain structure issues.

These were both really frustrating situations that taught me so much about asking even more specific questions and trusting myself to say, "No" when things feel off regardless of what the experts say. They taught me to be clear about what and why we are doing the things we are doing. If only I had known then what I now know we would have saved ourselves a lot of money and stress.

Margaret-ism
Pressing the Override Button

One of the things that I think is really important, and also really challenging at times, is to listen to and trust what we know to be true for us, our children and our families. As we navigate a lot of unknowns in parenting it can feel reassuring to do what someone tells us is best. Those "someones" can be experts in their field or other parents who experience similar unknowns, differences or challenges. While reassuring, sometimes it results in us pressing the "override button," allowing a course of action to occur or continue even though something doesn't feel right or best for your particular situation.

So, what sort of situations might we encounter in which we are tempted to hit the button that overrides our discomforts, hesitancies and doubts?

- Continuing an "off the shelf, one size fits all" therapy program that seems inappropriate for your child's specific needs.
- Keeping your child in a school that clearly is not meeting his needs because you've been told he needs the socializing influence of other kids.
- Continuing the employment of an inattentive caregiver who is not really helping your child because you feel guilty about letting them go.

Parenting isn't always easy and the path isn't always clear.

We may press the override button because we are tired or because there aren't other options and we want them to learn and grow.

We may press the override button because we are people pleasers and don't want to offend, hurt or dismiss what someone else shares with us.

We may press the override button because we've been convinced that the expert recommended by a trusted friend knows better than we do about what's best for our child.

To this all I say...

- We know our children best.
- We are the experts of our children.
- We are their team leaders.

With these things in mind, we can absolutely consult the advice of experts and other parents who are on similar parenting journeys AND filter that advice with what we know about our children. We can take that into consideration when we are making choices about services, schools and caregivers.

If you relate to pressing the override button, you are not alone! What can be helpful is to become aware of times when you did this and to get curious about why you did it. For me personally, it was about people pleasing and also assuming the experts knew best. I wanted people to like me and I wanted to look like a good mom. Not surprisingly, none of these self-serving motivations that caused me to press the override button led to better outcomes for me, my child or our family.

Noticing when I want to press it and pausing to get clear about my intention and motivation (my what and my why), tap a reservoir of power and clarity that allow me to make choices that are better aligned with who my child is in the present moment and what forms of support are the most appropriate for the situation. I don't know about you but for me, that far outweighs any benefit I may receive from getting approval from others.

Calling In the Archetypes

Situations where you feel judgment are the perfect times to play with the four archetypes I mentioned earlier...

- **Monarch (Queen/King), Elder** - Big picture vision and using past experiences and knowledge to guide decision making
- **Child** - Curiosity and play
- **Warrior** - Details, focused energy and boundary setting

- **Teacher/Community Builder** - Educating, supporting and celebrating

It can be really helpful to get curious about the particular strengths and energies each archetype can bring to challenging situations. The empowering tools they offer can turn uncomfortable, chaotic experiences into less stressful, more satisfying learning experiences.

Let's take, as an illustration, the stressful situation I mentioned earlier where my son is making loud, mucus-clearing sounds in a restaurant full of people...clearly a situation in which I was sure our fellow diners were judging both me and my son. How might I approach that situation from the perspective of these four archetypes?

Using the big picture/experiential wisdom of the Monarch/Elder, I might consider why he is engaging in this behavior at this time.

- My child could be anxious.
- He could be picking up on the funky energy of others around us which tends to cause him to make these noises.
- It could be an environment that is overwhelming his sensory system.

Tapping into the curiosity of the Child archetype can allow me to try different things to see if there is anything I can do to influence a difficult situation like this.

- I could distract him or try to make him feel more comfortable.
- We could go for a walk to the bathroom or see if we could move tables.
- It might also help me to determine if those judging us are worth my energy.

The Warrior is great at setting boundaries and this can happen in lots of different ways.

- I can set a boundary for myself by not giving my attention to what the others around us are doing, even if they give us a dirty look.
- It could be setting a boundary with them by staring right back without apology.

The Teacher/Community Builder can be helpful in determining who is on our "team" and who is not.

- If the other people around us feel kind, loving, open to learning and accepting, I might find a simple way to let them know that I'm doing the best I can.
- Do all I can to bring my focus into the small circle of me and my son and not give a s#!t about what other people think.

The more you can remain in the archetypal energy that supports clarity about what actually matters in the moment, the more you can tap into your experience and wisdom in order to trust what you know about your child.

I strongly encourage you to play with this in situations that aren't filled with judgment, like solo trips to the store. When I began playing with this, it was in grocery stores and Target trips that I would take alone.

I would check in with my Queen to see what the big picture was for this shopping trip, usually to get groceries or items that are needed for meals or for our home.

I would then check in with my Warrior to create a list to keep me focused and not forget items.

From there I would enlist my Child to see how to make this most pleasurable which usually meant starting the stopwatch on my clock app in order to see how fast I could get in and out OR I could enjoy my alone time while also listening to my favorite music or podcasts.

My Community Builder/Teacher was encouraging me to use what I know and to celebrate and enjoy the time I had as well as the fact that I was doing something to care for myself and my family.

Example:

My son hated when I would see someone I knew while we were grocery shopping and I grew to not like it as well because he would yell things like, "Stop talking!" and the other person never seemed to pick up on the cues that this wasn't a good time to catch up on our lives. I would tell him that it would only be a minute but it always ended up being more.

Rather than worrying about them judging me and my son for his lack of patience during these times, I eventually realized I needed a bit of Monarch/Elder and Warrior energy during these situations.

My Monarch/Elder gave me permission to not feel like I needed to have these conversations at that moment in time and used my Warrior to set some boundaries by setting a timer and telling them I needed to move on when the timer went off.

This made my son feel much less anxious about the potential of a never-ending conversation between mom and her friend.

I also made a point of reaching out to them and finding a time where we could have lunch or a phone call to catch up which made my Community Builder/Teacher happy.

Playing with this in situations we frequently find ourselves can help to build new patterns so that when you find yourself in a challenging situation where people are judging, or you think that they are, it feels more comfortable to immediately empower yourself to tap into each of these archetypal energies in order to be as effective and efficient as possible in supporting you and your child with your valuable energy and attention.

Now that you have greater awareness of what might come up for you with regards to control and judgment, let's explore the importance of curiosity and feedback in determining what might be underneath those challenging situations that involve strong emotional reactions, like meltdowns, tantrums, power struggles, resistance, anxiety, avoidance, etc.

Chapter Fourteen

Curiosity, Feedback and the Three Questions

A significant shift in empowering yourself along the way of this hero's journey in parenting can happen when you are able to become more of an observer of what is going on with you, your child, those around you or situations as a whole. This ability requires you to toggle back and forth between zooming out and zooming in.

Now we'll learn to expand on that skill, combining it with the use of intention and curiosity to become the ultimate observer. Becoming an observer allows you to gather feedback and gathering feedback is the first step to empowering yourself and your ability to parent.

Diving Deeper into Curiosity and Feedback

As I have been trying to shine a light on obstacles that might present themselves to you, I also hope that there has been something sparked inside of you - a renewed sense of curiosity. While the initial desire might be to have a set plan to follow, curiosity is what is actually the most helpful in the constant unknowns and unexpecteds of parenting.

Curiosity is a tool that can make a significant impact in how you are perceiving your current circumstances. It can also help you shift your approach and the experience of what comes next. While the Warrior prefers the "blinders on" approach in order to keep things focused and maintain an illusion of control, curiosity takes those blinders off.

Once the blinders come off, all sorts of possibilities appear as you are able to zoom out. Zooming out gives you a different perspective from lots of different angles. Zooming back in helps you to sort out your options to better inform decision making.

Your Monarch/Elder archetype *loves* approaching things from a zoomed out or big picture perspective. This is how they can act as a guiding force and inform the other archetypes of what they need to do so all are on the same page in order to support you in supporting your child. This allows you to have clarity of vision along with purposeful action and this shift feels so good!!

Curiosity is something that we all have in childhood and it helps us learn and grow by looking at everything as simply feedback. *This worked. This didn't. Let me play with this and see what happens.*

These three questions were introduced when I mentioned the difference between "work" and "play" and utilizing the Child archetype to be creative with problem solving. Let's explore them a bit more to see how they can truly help us in parenting as a clarity building force if we embrace them.

The Three Questions

1 - What's working?

All too often, what we know works or what has worked in the past, gets forgotten. There is a ton that we know that works for us, for our children, for our families, even if it was one time a few years ago! Let's bring those things to the forefront in order to use them to our advantage!!

2 - What's not working?

This question usually gets all of our attention in a negative way. But if we can get curious about what is not working in a particular situation, it doesn't have to be a negative experience. And, we might not have to toss everything we are doing out the window and start from scratch! There could be just one little piece of the equation that gets us off track. Investigating what that might be can help us to get back on track much faster.

3 - What is something I/we can do differently to see if it gets us closer to our intention?

This is all about using what you learned from the previous two questions to brainstorm different things to try in order to support you, your child and your family. This is the "Attention" part of my TIANT Process.

Most of the time our brains tend to overlook what IS working in our lives. These three simple questions created a powerful shift in my energy because they required my Storyteller to use my creative thinking mind in a different way. The things that I noticed became information rather than a negative thought, story or judgment. It was all quite freeing and more like working on a puzzle. I could figure it out without putting pressure on myself or my child to resolve it correctly on the first try!

I also became more aware of what things went well and I made sure to tuck those away for the future. This inquiry into what worked helped me gather information rather than constantly wasting time and energy by reinventing the wheel. As I gathered more information and a deeper understanding of what would be helpful for us all, the exhaustion I had been feeling for years lifted.

The Three Questions in Action

My son is a visual learner/processor, he does best when things are put in writing. There are times when I will tell him to do something ("telling" is the key here, as that's good for an auditory learner/processor but not so much for a visual one!)

and it doesn't get done. When I can remember what I know works for him, i.e. putting it in writing so he can see it, the whole experience goes much smoother.

Before I learned to use the three questions, my energy and focus would be on the fact that he hadn't done what I had asked and our interaction would be dominated by my frustration and annoyance. However, by using the knowledge gathered during the "What's Working?" phase of the three questions, I can avoid the negative thoughts and distancing negative emotions they elicit while connecting with my son more supportively and effectively. Now, we use lots of checklists and text messages. This way, he has a visual to refer back to, things usually get done and I feel more ease.

When things don't go well, these questions help me to not beat myself up. Rather than telling myself all sorts of stories, like how I am a bad parent or how everyone else seems to know what to do, I now get curious about the reality of the situation. From there, I can more clearly see what I could do differently (either in the moment or in the future) to influence the situation in order to create more of what I was intending.

These three questions significantly transformed my parenting experience. Rather than looking at a meltdown, tantrum, frustrations, or annoyances as situations that simply sucked, I began to see them as situations that were providing me with important feedback. I could tease things out, using curiosity to look into all of the parts and pieces of the situation. I like to look at it as rewinding a scene in a movie, in order to create more awareness of what was actually going on. It is all just feedback after all in order to make different choices the next time!

Why do we lose our sense of curiosity? I think that beginning in elementary school, kids begin to experience feelings of anxiety about not getting something right or things not working out the way they want them to. As a consequence, they become reluctant to follow their curiosity into the unknown. Perhaps they begin to feel that asking a lot of questions is not the way to gain the approval of the teacher or their peers. Or, perhaps their family simply does not value curiosity and thinking outside the box.

This can continue as we take on the responsibilities of adulthood and the doubts, uncertainties and unknowns become more threatening to our ego. As adults, we seem more likely to believe that our curiosity might reveal something we didn't want to know (or should already have known). And if that is the case, again as busy adults trying to keep our train on the rails, we would likely feel a grudging responsibility to do something with that information. Even worse, if we chose to ignore what we learned by being curious, we would be saddled with feelings of guilt and incompetence. Abandoning our curiosity could be a way of avoiding adding more responsibilities to our adult lives.

Whatever the reason or whenever our curious tendencies get questioned, the part of ourselves that craves acceptance begins to steer us towards what seems safer, following laid out paths and/or what others tell us we "should" do. Our decisions go from a curiosity driven perspective of experimentation and a "let's see what happens" attitude to ones more aligned with "I cannot risk failure so it's best to stay with what is known."

One of the things that I believe the children of those of us on this hero's journey in parenting are here to teach us is to recognize when our ego is leading, that there is no known and that curiosity is incredibly helpful and freeing for all of those involved. This requires openness, vulnerability and a willingness to look at things that don't go as expected as information to help guide us in the future. If you play with this, you will begin to feel that shift into a more calm and empowered energy. Your child will feel this as well.

Part Four Conclusion: Summary, Key Concepts and Power Questions

Summary:

Control and judgment are Hindering Forces that hold you back from feeling ease, peace and joy in parenting. They create false stories (thanks to the Storyteller) that lead to filtering experiences and interactions through a lens that creates a great deal of tension. While there is very little in your life that can be controlled, we can control our responses and reactions to these stories...even if they involve judgment.

Key Concepts:

- Control and the Roles of the Storyteller, Battle Ready Bodyguard and the Guardian of Your Heart
- TIANT Process
- Relinquishing Control and Building Your Support Network
- Shadow Payoffs
- Judgment Storm in Parenting - Self, Child, Others
- Radar Tool
- Experts Aren't Always the Experts of Your Child

- Pressing the Override Button
- Bringing in the Archetypes When Feeling Judged
- Curiosity, Feedback and the Three Questions

Power Questions:

- What is causing me tension?
- What is my intention?
- What attention can I give to that intention?
- What expectation do I need to let go of in order to have no (or less) tension?
- What is the shadow payoff I'm getting for doing this or being this way?
- Byron Katie's Question - Whose business am I in?
- What am I making it mean?
- Who am I handing my power over to?
- Who becomes more important than what I know?
- Whose opinion becomes more significant than my child?
- What am I noticing?
- What is working?
- What is not working?
- What is one thing I can do differently?

PART FIVE

Stormy Times of Parenting - Meltdowns and Tatrums

You've been wandering on this hero's journey in parenting, hopefully getting to know more about yourself with regards to your thoughts, body and emotions. You might be feeling pretty strong when all of a sudden...BAM!

Something in the air shifts, energies get big and your child starts having some very strong emotions. This could come in the form of anger, anxiety or shutting down. This can look like yelling, hitting, spitting, throwing, running or hiding. This feels incredibly intense and more than anything, you just want it to stop.

I get it. I tried all I could to stop my son's strong emotions and the behaviors associated with them. I looked at my son's strong emotions as an out of control fire that had to be extinguished. I approached him as though I had a fire extinguisher in my hand, hosing down the emotions with equally strong emotional energy. What I wasn't looking at, and taking into consideration, were the things that caused the strong feelings in the first place.

Hosing down my son's emotions was not working for either of us. In fact, it only made things worse. Once I became aware of this, I began to zoom out and get curious about what might actually be happening and wow, was there a treasure trove of information to explain the feedback I was getting in the form of those emotions.

This certainly did not happen overnight and it took lots of pauses, deep breaths, patience and learning how to be okay in the moment with someone who was feeling strong emotions. This all led to some major changes within me that helped tremendously during these unexpected and challenging times. It also made me extremely curious about what was actually going on and I learned some common causes.

Common Causes for Meltdowns and Tantrums

Over the years of personal and professional experience, I have been tracking underlying causes for meltdowns and tantrums and I've boiled them down to the following:

- Sensory Overload
- Emotional Regulation Challenges
- Embarrassment
- Chronological Age vs Development Age
- Learning Stage Exhaustion
- Desire to Control and Testing Boundaries
- The Need to Close an Open Loop

> Other underlying causes can be PDA (Pervasive Desire for Autonomy or Pathological Demand Avoidance) or Executive Functioning Challenges. I am not an expert in either of these so if you want to learn more, Dr. Melissa Neff has knowledge and experience in PDA and Seth Perler is an Executive Functioning expert and both have done episodes with Debbie Reber on the TiLT Parenting Podcast about these topics.

I find that having a mental list of the possible causes or triggers can make a huge difference in how I approach the situation because so often what we might assume is going on based on the surface behaviors is rarely what is actually going on. Using the question *"What is actually going on?"* is extremely helpful here, too.

I love this question because it is never not helpful. It always works to shift my attention into noticing and observer mode, even if just for a few seconds.

Let's explore each of these potential underlying causes in greater detail so you know what to be on the lookout for. I will also share some ideas on what you can do to support yourself and your child during these challenging times when they occur.

Chapter Fifteen

Underlying Cause: Sensory Overload

Sensory input comes in from sights, sounds, smells, tastes, feeling, touch, texture and energy. If your child has a sensitive sensory system or if they have sensory processing challenges (SPD - sensory processing disorder), which are common among neurodivergent individuals, normal sounds, smells or textures can become too much for the child to manage.

My son would frequently plug his ears in order to cut off his sense of sound when in a new environment or busy situation. He was doing this because the sensory information he was taking in was too intense for him. Plugging his ears was his way of being able to adjust, regulate and soothe himself when he couldn't control the volume of things around him. Other people have difficulty with tastes, smells or the feeling of things against their skin.

I view our sensory system like dials on a stereo system that control the volume, bass, treble, balance, etc. and I imagine that each of the senses is its own dial. When someone has a sensitive sensory processing system, they might not be able to automatically adjust the "dial" up or down in order to automatically regulate themselves. Occupational therapy and learning strategies to support them in learning how to be aware of their "dials" can make a big difference.

Mindfulness around your child's particular sensitivities can also help you have strategies in your back pocket to support them when sensory overload occurs. This is particularly helpful to know as environments that our children are frequently placed in can exacerbate their sensitivities, like the lunchroom or gymnasium where the smells, sounds and energy can be challenging to navigate.

> Having monitored these places while teaching, I can attest that they can be intense for people who DON"T have sensory regulation challenges.

Some strategies we have used to help our son include:

- Noise canceling headphones or earbuds with apps like White Noise, Calm, or BrainWave in order to buffer noises that might agitate him.
- Being mindful of the food that we are cooking, allowing him to eat his food somewhere else if our food has a smell that is too strong for him.
- Making changes with regards to perfume, cologne and candles. He likes some scents or smells and others are too strong. I used to carry cotton balls

scented with essential oils (lavender and balsam fir were his favorites) in a plastic bag for times when we were out and he felt anxious or if something or if someone had a strong smell.

A lot of our children have heightened energetic sensitivities and being aware of the energy of different people and spaces is something that is rarely discussed but can be really helpful because it can be another underlying cause for strong emotional responses or reactions.

If the energy of the space or people is intense, we try to have timeouts in quiet areas. This might even be necessary at family gatherings or birthday parties where there are a lot of people. You might go into these experiences thinking that your children will love these activities because they are excited beforehand AND these can be prime situations to ramp them up, cause sensory overload, resulting in a meltdown.

Common places where things can be particularly overwhelming are kitchens, playgrounds, other people's houses, lunchrooms, airports, malls, theme/amusement parks, etc. The next time you are in an airport, take a minute and check in with all of your senses, including noticing the energy around you. When I do this, I can sense a lot of nervous, frantic and excited energy in addition to the smells of all of the different restaurants in the food court, the beeping of carts, announcements being made, etc. It is a lot to take in!

While you cannot do anything to control the intense sensory or energetic experiences of these different places, awareness can help change how you approach them. It can also increase compassion and understanding of what is actually going on when strong responses appear. You can become more mindful of the spaces in which your child might be reaching their toleration limit and you can adjust or support them with helpful strategies that have worked in the past.

> I used to call my son an emotional energy BS detector because I could tell from how he interacted with someone whether or not they felt safe to him. It was sometimes subtle with him just walking past a caregiver in order to spin cups on the table at the kids club at our gym or a sudden escalation of rigidity or yelling when waiting in line to get onto an airplane. As stated above, observing this allowed me to have a better understanding of what might actually be going on which could help me to do what I could to calm him as opposed to placing my own energy and attention on the rigidity or yelling.

Chapter Sixteen

Underlying Cause: Emotional Regulation Challenges

Managing a child's emotions can be challenging as emotions can come on fast and furious. Their reactions and emotions might not always seem logical or rational, unless we know all that was going on with our child and the situation beforehand. Remember that an emotional outburst —whether verbally or physically— is an inability to regulate emotions. So the emotions come out without a filter. This doesn't mean it's fun, it just helps to view it from a different perspective, one where you don't feel like a metaphorical (or an actual) punching bag.

It has helped me think of my son's meltdowns and tantrums as PMS-ing. Strong emotional energy seemingly comes out of nowhere and the next thing I know, I'm wanting to pick a fight with my husband so I can have someone else to engage in this unstable energy with me. Again, it's not necessarily logical or rational. It doesn't make sense when you're not the one experiencing these emotions and can be extremely uncomfortable for all involved, rarely leaving anyone feeling any better until the emotional energy dissipates.

While PMS is the result of shifting hormone levels, in my experience, a child experiencing strong emotions usually has some common underlying causes. This can be feelings of embarrassment, disappointment, frustration or a lack of control. Shifting hormones during puberty can also be a contributing factor.

When your child expresses intense emotion in public, it can cause people around them to feel uncomfortable and want it to stop because it looks and feels different from what they know. They can get upset and have equally intense reactions that usually involve either trying to assert some form of judgmental look or comment to try to control, which does nothing to help the situation.

It would be wonderful if people could realize that in those moments, the child's strong emotions are the result of emotional regulation challenges. They often stem from underlying factors like sensory processing, unclosed loops of expectation, their own desire to control, etc. It would be better if others could be more compassionate and understand that there is probably something more going on than meets the eye that is causing the behaviors that look different from what they are accustomed to in social situations.

But wishing and hoping for that is oftentimes unrealistic and, ultimately, a waste of your time and energy. Instead, in these sorts of public situations, the best approach as a parent is to ignore as much as possible the uninformed negative reactions of others and use your own informed understanding of what your child is currently experiencing to avoid the "power and control" intervention that only tends to make the situation worse.

> During times like this I envision a target and know that I have to be at the center and my child is the first ring and that is all that matters. Family and friends might be on the next few rings and strangers on rings that are farthest from the center. The amount of energy and attention each ring gets diminishes the farther out they are and if that makes those in outer rings feel uncomfortable, too bad. You need to place your energy and attention on doing what is best for you and your child during challenging times.

There are things you can do to support your child and encourage better ways of managing their emotions once things return to baseline. However, when emotions are running high, engaging in an emotional power struggle with them is not helpful and usually leaves everyone feeling like crap.

> Baseline occurs when emotions have died down and we are all back to a more calm and regulated state of being.

Let's play with a metaphor tool that always helps me during these times...

Margaret's Fire Metaphor Tool

Imagine that the strong emotion your child is experiencing and expressing is like a fire in a fire pit or fireplace. What do I notice? What happens to the raging fire when your best attempt to put it out involves throwing rationalizing or problem solving strategies at it? What happens when your fire extinguisher is spraying anxious energy in the form of frenetic movements and verbalizations? But what happens to the fire if you press the pause button, take a few deep breaths, and approach the fire with a calm, and maybe even curious, energy.

Viewing it in this way and asking myself these sorts of questions has helped me become more of an observer, which is actually helpful. When I approach things this way, I learn so much about what I was doing that wasn't productive and am able to see what I could do differently to be more effective.

I realized that meeting their intense emotional energy with equally intense emotional energy simply adds oxygen or fuel to the fire that, more often than not, causes it to flare up. Slowing down, taking deep breaths, not engaging or getting tangled up in it (while still keeping them and others safe) is the opposite of not adding fuel to the fire. Doing this might feel counterproductive and uncomfortable but it actually allows their emotional "fire" to die down faster.

I've learned that sometimes I forget and accidentally add another log (or some more kindling) to his fire by raising my voice, using a strong tone or increasing my energy. This is all fuel for his fire. Good to know because once I'm aware of this, I can press pause, take some more deep breaths and get back to remembering what I know is actually helpful...NOT getting tangled up in his strong energy by engaging with equally strong emotions or energy.

It's always a great reminder that meltdowns and tantrums are often coming from an inability to process and regulate emotions. This can significantly impact interactions with your child because you will most likely be more patient, compassionate and empathetic with them...and yourself.

If you need something to say, try using a mantra like, "I will help you when your body is calm." This can help because it can give you some time and space to calm down and remind you not to engage in verbal entanglements that many of our children are brilliant at. Many times it feels like they are future attorneys in training, documenting, remembering and using our words to support their case. It also lets the child know that you will help them, but cannot do so until they are calm.

> They might not like this but remember that most of the time they are looking for or wanting fuel for their fire. Not giving it to them might bother them but is better than the outcomes of engaging and fueling.

This particular mantra came to me years ago during a situation with my son. He was upset about something not working the way he wanted it to work and was feeling very strong emotions. This led to his body being dysregulated and him wanting to be physical with me.

When he was younger, I would hold him or ride this out with him in a room together. However, he was now as big as me, which made this option not the safest for me.

I had tried all I could to figure out how to help him. I didn't want to be on the receiving end of any hitting or kicking and I could sense this was about to start. It got to a point where I knew I needed to calm myself before I could do anything more so I went into my room and sat against the locked door. I needed a time out and I told him so. He started banging on the door. I took a deep breath and said, "I will help you when your body is calm."

That is the only thing I allowed myself to say to him. After about five minutes of him trying to get me to make promises I couldn't keep, combined with banging on the door, he calmed. I opened the door and he started again. I calmly said, "I can only help you when your body is calm." It took a while for the strong emotions to pass because he was disappointed. He thought he could get me engaged in his strong emotions and I refused.

While this lasted a while, his emotions passed much quicker than they would have had I gotten tangled up in his energy - meeting it with my own equally intense energy which is what worked for my parents when I was growing up. This used to happen all of the time, with miserable results, before I understood the power of untangling and creating space!

You may worry that you are minimizing your child's experience or frustration when you aren't engaging with their emotions.

But in my experience, it is quite the opposite. Not a lot can be accomplished when someone isn't calm and/or ready for help. This may require some repatterning if your child is used to you engaging, but I am living proof that it can be done!

Chapter Seventeen

Underlying Cause: Embarrassment

Ah...embarrassment. One of the least talked about challenges we face as human beings because it requires a great deal of humility and vulnerability. Thank you Brene Brown for bringing vulnerability out of the shadows and into the light! Only when there is awareness around something can change happen. Back when I was starting my hero's journey in parenting, I never heard anyone talking about embarrassment, how it shows up with our children and most importantly, what we as parents can do to support them when they are feeling this way.

If no one was talking about this back then, how did I get here? Well, it was 2009, I was prepping for dinner and my son was having a snack at the counter when he accidentally spilled his water. All of a sudden, he got down from the barstool, tipped it over and began scanning the area, looking for what else he could tip over.

I was in the process of getting a towel to help him wipe up the water when he did this. It was not like him at all to respond this way and I got curious about why he would be doing these things. What popped up in my mind and also surprised me a bit was this question, "Could he be embarrassed?" My initial response was, "No way! It's just me. Why would he be embarrassed in front of me?" But I bypassed my thought and asked him if he was embarrassed.

He immediately replied, "Yes. I am never going to spill my water again. I hate when things happen that I don't mean to do."

This awareness changed my approach to the tipped over chairs completely. Had I not known why he was doing this, I would have thought that he was just being a turd. But the energy of this conversation was completely different, supportive and without shaming because I approached it considering the underlying cause.

I proceeded to tell him that everyone spills things, it's no big deal. Things like this happen to me all of the time. I gave him a towel and helped him wipe it up, helped him pick up the chair and helped him refill his cup.

If I had gotten angry at him for tipping the chair, I would have been addressing the wrong trigger. We talked about how knocking things over or breaking things intentionally when we are upset or embarrassed doesn't fix anything and just creates more to deal with. But the energy of this conversation was completely different, supportive and without shaming because I approached it considering the underlying cause.

Embarrassment is certainly a part of emotional regulation and it shows up in shadowy ways, like aggression or defensiveness when someone gets caught doing something wrong. It can also show up as strong emotions when the child becomes aware that they didn't do something "right" or as "good" as someone else. (Parents of perfectionists, I'm talking to you!)

The simple recognition that a behavior is coming from a place of embarrassment can change the conversation as well as the underlying emotions of a situation. Reframing the incident as a basic fact of life, sometimes accidents happen, things don't go the way we plan and we aren't always the "best" at something. These honest reframes can help your child feel more comfortable in navigating and regulating their own emotions in the future.

I strongly encourage you to point out the times that things don't go well or play out as planned for you. Share your frustration and what you are going to do to get back on track. Laugh at yourself or the outcome in order to model for them that this is all part of being a human being who is meant to learn and grow.

I just did this a few days ago when I was filling a new dog food dispenser, pouring the dog food in the top of the canister while also forgetting that there was a dispenser hole in the bottom so when I lifted it off of the counter, dog food went everywhere! Definitely unexpected and I invited my son into the laundry room to see the mess I had made while also allowing him to see me laughing at myself for forgetting something so basic, like the design of this new item.

Things don't always go perfectly AND you have a choice in what you make it mean, especially about yourself.

Chapter Eighteen

Underlying Cause: Chronological Age vs. Developmental Age

As long as the earth's journey around the sun doesn't change dramatically, our chronological age is fixed from the date of our birth. This is not the case with developmental age. One's developmental age can change depending on the situation, sometimes moment to moment. Understanding and staying aware of this fact has been tremendously helpful for me as a parent and has helped my clients to better meet their child where they are based on a simple curiosity utilizing the question...

How old is my child at this moment?

> It's not just my child by the way. I might be 49 years old but there are times when I just want to play loud music, drive with my windows down while singing at the top of my lungs and not want to do any adulting activities...much like a 16 year old. Turns out, it's not just me and I'm sure

you've witnessed adults acting like children throwing tantrums over things like delayed or canceled flights. Sure those are not ideal, but like I tell my son in situations like this, "We cannot control things like weather, mechanical issues or lack of flight crew. We can take some deep breaths to see if there is anything we can do and if not, find a way to make the best of the situation we are in."

We all have these moments and the awareness that our child's developmental age can shift moment to moment can make a big difference as a parent.

Example:

My son was 7 years old and he had done something that I felt was timeout worthy despite knowing that historically timeouts never went well for us. They always ended with me getting more upset because he hated being put in his room alone so he'd throw things all over his room and then when it was over, I would try to get him to clean up the mess he made, because, you know, "consequences for actions," which sent us into more strong emotions that meant that the initial 5 minute timeout became an hour long ordeal. Not a great cycle to be in and it clearly wasn't working.

When I got curious about why I was doing this, my Storyteller pulled out of its book of internal rules and created a thought that there "should" be consequences for what he was doing. And this consequence needed to look a certain way, in particular, the way it looked when I was growing up and from what I knew from other parents.

On that particular day, I realized my approach to this was completely wrong, consequences and all! I wanted to put him in his room for a time-out because that is what I thought I "should" do. Instead, I began to get curious about why it never worked. I looked at him and at that moment, he certainly didn't feel like a 7 year old to me. He was behaving more like a 3 year old. And wouldn't you know it, what he had done certainly aligned with what a 3 year old would have done. I paused and asked myself, "How would I have handled this when he was 3?"

It was then that I realized that I would have handled it in several different ways.

I would have sat with him during the time out rather than putting him in his room alone because this always led to another battle. Why? Despite other parents being able to put their kids in their rooms for time outs at his chronological age, he knew what I didn't - he was not ready for it. He didn't understand why he needed to be isolated from me during those times. He couldn't connect what he had done 5 minutes ago with the response I had and the consequence I was giving.

As we sat, I would have tried to calm myself by taking deep breaths and not talking. During times like these, all parties involved usually have heightened energy. Taking some deep breaths, calming down and moving slower can be incredibly helpful.

The amount of time for the time-out would have been much less.

I wouldn't have had all of the stories circling in my mind about why he shouldn't have done what he did.

Knowing I had nothing to lose, I tried those very things.

I pulled two kitchen chairs in front of the microwave and set the timer for 3 minutes. I told him if he got up, I would reset it. He got up a few times and we probably sat there for 10 minutes total. (Looking back, I would have set it for much less basing it on my intention, which was for his body to calm, but since this was the first time trying this new strategy, we lived and I learned.)

This new way of supporting my child in learning and growing worked so much better because I was meeting him where he was developmentally. I was no longer beating my head against the wall trying to place expectations on him based on his chronological age.

From that day on, one of my favorite questions to ask when my son, or anyone for that matter, is having strong emotions is...

How old is this individual developmentally right now?

This question is HUGE because it puts our Storyteller to work gathering relevant information rather than gathering shaming stories. With our children, quite often their developmental age - their ability to regulate their emotions, their motor skills, their social skills, etc. - is much younger than their chronological age.

It can also be very tricky because you may have a child who one minute is discussing a very advanced topic for their age, like coding, physics or the meaning of life, and the next minute they are having a meltdown because there is a parsley speck on their pasta.

When your child is having a meltdown or tantrum, ask yourself the question, "How old is my child developmentally right now?" Asking this can help you meet them where they are so you can use strategies that are helpful at the appropriate developmental age.

This is also helpful to consider because oftentimes people expect others to behave in ways that are consistent with their chronological age which can lead to a lot of tension if the individual may not be developmentally capable of meeting those expectations.

This is part of emotional regulation and again, realizing that they cannot control this can help you in meeting them where they are in the moment while supporting them without judgment or expectations.

Chapter Nineteen

Underlying Cause: Learning Stage Exhaustion

I was introduced to many different learning stage models during my education studies at the University of Dayton and was reintroduced to the "Four Stages of Competence" during my nature-based coach training; however, it wasn't until parenting my son that I realized the significant role they play in emotional regulation for children.

The deeper I dove into these stages, the more I realized how important the awareness of them helps in supporting my child and the children of my clients. It has been an incredibly helpful perspective around another underlying cause of strong emotions and challenging times.

The "Four Stages of Competence" are:

- **Unconscious Incompetence** - when you don't know that you don't know something
- **Conscious Incompetence** - when you are aware that you don't know something or know how to do something but are working on learning it
- **Conscious Competence** - you know something or know how to do something but still have to think about it
- **Unconscious Competence** - you know something or know how to do something and don't have to even think about it

---

In order to have this make more sense, I love to compare this to driving a car. When you were little, you were most likely in the "unconscious incompetence" stage about what was happening in the driver's seat. Maybe you crawled into the driver's seat, held the steering wheel, and believed you were driving the car but had it been turned on and started moving, regardless of how often you were driven around, you didn't know what to do.

When you grew older and got behind the wheel for the first time, you were probably quite aware that you didn't really know what to do to actually make the car go and follow the laws, so you were "consciously incompetent" and if you wanted to know how to drive, you realized you had to learn somehow.

Whatever form of driver's ed you pursued, you got more experience by actually driving around and therefore, you became "consciously competent." While you had a better sense of what needed to happen when you sat down, you were still learning the rules of the road and had to spend energy focusing on what needed to happen, like where your hands were on the steering wheel, what your feet were doing and what your eyes needed to pay attention to.

You now are most likely in the stage of "unconscious competence" when driving, not having to spend a good deal of energy on all of the details for what needs to happen in order to get from point A to point B, other than knowing where you are going and having directions if necessary.

Hopefully this example gives you a basic framework of these "Four Stages of Competence."

Let's now think about how these stages apply to children who are on their own developmental timelines...especially when they hit ages 7-10 when awareness of differences between themselves and others seems to heighten.

Our children spend a majority of the time, especially during organized activities like school and sports teams, doing lessons or activities that introduce a new concept, provide opportunities to practice that new concept, gain competence in that concept and then, BAM!, it is back to learning the next new thing, which means they are constantly toggling back and forth between conscious incompetence and conscious competence.

> This is not limited to just academics, but can occur with building fine and gross motor skills, emotional development, social interactions, executive functioning, sensory experiences, basically anything that pushes the edge of what they are able to do and/or handle.

School, therapy and organized activities all require a lot of mental, emotional and possibly physical energy. Having to spend a good deal of their energy in those ways (toggling between conscious incompetence and conscious competence) means they don't get a lot of opportunities to feel truly competent or spend time enjoying well-learned activities that require minimal mental or physical energy (areas of unconscious competence).

Trying to achieve competence at any task takes effort, that is to say it removes energy from our limited reservoir. Moving through a series of learning challenges can eventually deplete energy resources. We've all experienced the demoralizing frustration of "hitting the wall", i.e. trying to accomplish something without the energy level necessary to meet the demands of the task. This situation of "hitting the wall" is a more common threat for children on their own developmental timeline (learning stage exhaustion) and, coupled with emotion management difficulties, can lead to somewhat predictable consequences---meltdowns, shutdowns, tantrums, etc. But for teachers who are not actively monitoring their students for this issue, these strong emotional responses to learning stage exhaustion may seem to come out of nowhere.

It is important to consider what might have been draining their energy could go beyond academics.

Getting through a PE class where it is loud, smelly while also needing to remember the rules of a game without any visuals, and then trying to do something that requires motor skills their body and brain may struggle with in order to move and bounce a ball without letting another child take it from them takes tremendous energy! Not surprising then when that child has a meltdown back in the classroom when the teacher introduces an activity that is challenging for them.

They aren't having a meltdown for no reason. Their metaphorical gas tank is empty! Curiosity around what the child might have been feeling prior to the meltdown can help the teacher press the pause button on their response to the meltdown and allow them to gather valuable information about what the child is actually experiencing. With less focus on the meltdown itself (which most often feels like shaming to the child), the teacher can look for ways to support the child by offering opportunities for the child to replenish their energy reservoir.

Awareness of learning stage exhaustion is also helpful for those times when they come home and take it out on those around them, like you or younger siblings! I have heard this time and again, parents are excited to see their children after school, and in less than a minute, they become a metaphorical punching bag as the child falls apart after holding it together all day. It is so easy to be blind-sided by this seemingly "out-of-nowhere" emotional assault and let ourselves be reflexively provoked into our own heated emotional response. But again, pausing to be curious about the underlying cause can allow you to sidestep the impending conflict and shift your perspective (and your energy) toward an outcome that keeps you connected to your child in a more supportive, satisfying way.

If this all resonates with you, it is important to provide time and opportunities for your child to enjoy their unique "unconscious competencies" as these are the activities that help them regulate their emotions, increase their confidence, refill their metaphorical energy tank and generally bolster their feelings of competence and confidence.

Allow Time for Your Child to Do What Comes Easy to Them, Their Unique Unconsciously Competent Activities!

I remember while growing up with three siblings ranging from toddler to teenager, I needed time alone after a day at school. My unique activities involved hitting a tennis ball against the garage door or riding my bike around our neighborhood while listening to my walkman.

My son's go-to activities are playing with his outdoor light sconces, wiring them up and changing bulbs. He also writes plays based on fictional characters doing things he has done, like celebrating holidays or visiting places he has gone.

We all have our own "flow" activities that we naturally gravitate towards and don't require a ton of energy, in fact they give us energy. Since most of these are done alone, we can have a sense of control around how we are doing them and therefore feel competent and confident.

(Insert Divider Line)

Possible "Unconsciously Competent" Activities (but certainly not limited to these things):

- Reading
- Singing
- Dancing
- Bouncing
- Swinging
- Climbing
- Baking or cooking
- Running or walking
- Swimming, showering, bathing
- Biking
- Puzzles
- Legos
- Building
- Writing
- Drawing, painting, coloring, etc.

- Knitting, crocheting, weaving, needlepoint or cross stitch, etc.
- Organizing
- Gaming or Screen time (You can create a structure or place limits on this if it becomes an issue with them getting off of screens to do other things OR if it ramps them up.)

Being conscious of your child's preferred activities can help you to be more intentional about making sure there is time for them to refuel so that they have the energy to better regulate themselves and their emotions.

Chapter Twenty

Underlying Cause: Desire to Control and Testing Boundaries

Feeling the need to control things isn't just something that we as parents face. Our children also have the desire to control things, especially during times of insecurity and uncertainty. Our children are not immune to wanting or needing to know what is going on and what they can do to influence what is happening in their own life.

Our children will also naturally want to test boundaries that others set for them in order to assert independence and also determine if boundaries are flexible or firm. This is a normal part of developmental learning and growing. Things become more complicated when a child's executive functioning and emotional regulation capabilities develop at a different rate and their efforts to exert independence are expressed through tantrums or meltdowns. This might be expected from a chronological two year old but is perceived quite differently when the child is chronologically older even if the child is developmentally two at that moment.

> It always helps me to consider the developmental age of the child during a tantrum or meltdown because I can play around with ways to support them at the developmental age they are rather than expecting them to be able to manage frustration, annoyance, irritation, etc. based on their chronological age. This becomes even more complicated when your child has an intellectual age much greater than their chronological age but handles frustrations at an age that is less than their chronological age.
>
> Example: A 10 year old child is coding a computer program like a 22 year old. There is a storm and the wifi connection goes offline. They start crying and throwing things around the room like a 3 year old. Same child, different developmental capabilities and ages all within a minute's time.

This can feel tricky as a parent. We want our children to feel like they have choices. We want them to learn how to be independent and how to navigate challenges and disappointments they will inevitably face as human beings AND when the balance begins to lean towards them needing to control and having tantrums in order to get what they want, leaving us walking on eggshells and moving heaven and earth to prevent tantrums, this does not feel good.

A tantrum is different from a meltdown. Its primary causes are not things like emotional regulation challenges, sensory processing challenges, anxiety, etc., but rather by the need to control. When your child is having a tantrum, they may try to get into a power struggle with you. Simply realizing that they are trying to get you to engage in the uncomfortable energy they are experiencing can make a big difference in how you feel and how you approach the situation.

One of the things I often get asked about is how to tell whether a child is having a meltdown or a tantrum. In order to determine this, pay close attention to what happens immediately after the strong emotional display. Have they been able to influence the situation in their favor? With a meltdown, there is usually not an immediate return to baseline as it takes time to move through the strong emotions felt.

One difference I have noticed is that when a tantrum ends, the child usually returns to baseline fairly quickly, content because they either got what they wanted or realized they weren't going to get it and ran out of energy fighting for it. Of course this isn't always the case but I've seen enough of both to have a good sense of which is which, and with some curiosity, you can start learning the specific differences with your child.

> I've seen children who smirk or look around to see if anyone noticed that they were able to get what they wanted by tantruming. I've seen confused parents who gave their child what they wanted and the child was still upset because they were having a meltdown and needed more time to calm down. Fascinating, isn't it?!

When you notice that your child is trying to control or is testing boundaries, this is a great time to bring your Child and Queen/King/Elder together, tap into curiosity by using the question, "What is actually going on here?" in order to help you to get the broader picture of the situation.

From there you can get clear on your intention for the moment. You can start to get curious and play around with what the child's intention might be, which can further guide you on how to approach the situation. I always find it fascinating to consider what they are wanting and why they are trying to control it.

Why are they testing or trying to control? The child might be testing boundaries or trying to control out of anxiety, fear of uncertainty, sensory or emotional regulation challenges, a response to too many demands placed upon them or out of an inability to delay gratification. They may also just want things to go their way.

> When anxiety takes over, there can be an intense desire to find some semblance of control. If an individual who is feeling anxious is pushed to do something that doesn't feel safe, it can elicit a meltdown in order to try to regain control. One common characteristic of an anxiety-induced meltdown is the irrational extremes the child will go to (whether it be unconstrained acts of physical or verbal aggression or refusal to act, the so-called "shutdown") in order to restore the feeling of being safe. Importantly, an anxiety-induced meltdown can be triggered as easily and

> quickly by an imagined threat as by a "real" threat. (I put "real" in quotation marks because even an imagined threat FEELS real to the individual experiencing it.)

When you have an awareness of possible reasons your child is having a meltdown, you can enlist your Warrior to use what you learned to come up with a plan to approach the situation in a way that will be more effective and efficient. It may also include setting some energetic boundaries for yourself so you don't get tangled up in their energy.

This can support your child in shifting away from the need or desire to control in ways that are more likely to be received by them. It can also help your child find ways to influence situations in a more kind and loving manner. Knowing the root cause of your child's desire to control, you are better able to support them.

Example:

My son starts to get into my personal space and will persistently ask me the same question when he is anxious about something. Recognizing this pattern helps me notice what is going on and do what I can to give myself what I need, usually a little bit of time and space to figure out what is causing his anxiety and what I can do to try and help him.

We experienced this very thing on a ski trip when he had given me his phone to hold while he went skiing with dad. There were a ton of things going on as they weren't planning on skiing that afternoon but our room wasn't ready so my husband decided it would be more fun to ski than wander aimlessly. Because I didn't want his phone to get lost, I placed it in my backpack which was being stored with the rest of our stuff, and then headed out with him to get his skis and boots from the rental place.

After he had what he needed, off they went and I sat down on an Adirondack chair in the village knowing that I had time to relax for a while before our room was ready. Once it was ready and they were done skiing, we were unpacking and my son asked me where his phone was. Ironically, despite my desire to keep his phone safe, I had totally forgotten that I had put it in my backpack and all I could think of was putting it where I usually put my phone...in my back pocket...which made me nervous that it had fallen out either at the ski rental shop while helping him to fit his boots or while sitting on the Adirondack chair.

My heart dropped because this is something very important to him and something he would not get over easily. He started ramping up his energy, telling me how he needed it and I began noticing myself ramping up because I was upset with myself and because I didn't want him to be upset. I told him I needed to think for a few minutes and put myself in the bathroom.

Within 30 seconds I remembered that I had put it in my backpack, grabbed it and brought it to him. I then told him that the only way I could have remembered that was by having some time and space to think.

While he will probably do the same thing the next time, what matters is that I know that I need this for myself in order to best problem solve and figure things out in order to support him. I have learned that his behavior is usually stemming from fear of uncertainty. When my son does this, I do what I can to give him appropriate information while also telling him that I need space in order to think. Having a better sense of the plan reduces his fear, though it doesn't eliminate it completely as shared above.

If the need for control is coming from my son's desire to want things to go his way, I would handle this with very different energy and attention.

Again, exploring the possible root causes of your child's behavior can help you help them find more kind, calm and loving ways to influence a situation, or even to plant the seed of what this can look like in order to cycle through things faster. They can then learn positive ways to take care of their needs and begin to establish independence.

Chapter Twenty-One

Underlying Cause: The Need to Close an Open Loop

When my son was younger, I discovered another underlying cause of meltdowns and tantrums that I call the "open loop." An open loop is exactly what it sounds like, something that has not been completed and in some people this can create a great deal of discomfort.

This became apparent when I had planned a playground visit that didn't happen due to rain. No amount of explaining to my son that we could go another time would suffice. The expectation, activity or task was not completed and this created a tremendous amount of anxiety for him.

I realized that this was an "open loop" for him and while we couldn't close it by going to the playground that day, I could try other ways of temporarily extending or closing it for him. I looked at the weather app with him and if there was a good day ahead, I put it on my calendar so that he knew I was serious about taking him to the playground. Closing the loop helped him to move on from any strong emotions and anxiety around his own thoughts, fears and dramaticizing that the playground visit was never going to happen...ever.

My son is a visual processor so when he could see the event scheduled on my calendar, he could mentally close the loop. I do similar things when we run out of favorite or preferred foods. I write it down or show him that I'm putting it on my next grocery delivery order.

If your child is an auditory processor, they may do best when you tell them things. So if you cannot tell them directly, leaving or sending them audio messages or calling/Facetime audio could be a good way for them to hear what needs to be conveyed, even if they are in the next room.

If your child is a kinesthetic processor, they most likely need to be actively engaged in something. You could make a countdown with post-it notes or have them physically cross dates off on a calendar to help them close their loop when things don't go as planned.

The next time your child has an expectation for something and then experiences some sort of disappointment or unexpected change in plans, take into consideration how they best process things - visually, auditorily or kinesthetically - and get curious about what could be done to help them close the loop. Being aware of this helps me to realize that there is more going on than the behavior or reaction that is taking place in front of me.

"When kids experience negative violations of some expectation (i.e. the disappointment and frustration that occurs when the expectation that something good is going to happen gets canceled or postponed), it does indeed create anxiety. This anxiety is a cue to press pause and get curious. What is it about this expectancy violation that causes anxiety? Some lines of research suggest that the anxiety is created because the expectancy violation is also a trust violation---the child's trust in the parent's ability to deliver on their promises is undermined, which is threatening to the child; and, second, the expectancy violation is threatening to the child's need to believe that events are controllable (the need for control that was previously covered). The interventions you've suggested to deal with a violated expectation are effective because they help to restore both trust and control by involving the child in how the violated expectation would be addressed and managed."

- William Webb, PhD

Chapter Twenty-Two

During and/or After a Meltdown or Tantrum (or Any Emotionally Charged Time)

Now that you've got some ideas on your radar for what could be going on during the meltdown or tantrum, let's explore some ways you can support yourself and your child.

Let's be honest...the initial desire during these emotionally charged and uncomfortable situations is almost always to make them stop as soon as possible. However, many of the approaches usually taken to do this only add fuel to the fire.

Many times parents and caregivers use methods that were used or modeled while they were growing up or do what they think they "should" be doing. I personally tried for years to do what I thought I "should" do or based on how I was parented and failed miserably each time because I was a rule-follower, a people pleasing child and my son was/is not.

In reflecting on how every child is different, I am grateful to have learned to approach meltdowns and tantrums from a different perspective. Utilizing the tools, questions and strategies that I've been sharing so far can be extremely helpful during these times. The tools that have been most helpful to me during tantrums and meltdowns include:

- Noticing.
- Curiosity.
- Intention.
- Questioning.

These four things have made a world of difference for me and my son because they shift the energy in a more productive and effective manner.

There is one additional thing that was crucial for me to understand in order to navigate my son's meltdowns, tantrums or anxiety - I had to learn to not engage in the intense energy of my child's meltdown and/or tantrum. Not engaging, as I mentioned earlier, usually means taking lots of deep breaths, slowing way down —almost to slow motion— and going into observer mode which allows for curiosity.

- *Is it an open loop?*
- *Is it a sensory or emotional regulation challenge?*
- *Are we getting into a power struggle?*
- *Are they tired/hungry/thirsty/exhausted of energy because the demands have been too much?*

If you do this, you will get a broader, more nuanced perspective on what is actually going on, not just what you "think" is going on. Trust me, there is a big difference!!

As previously mentioned, I also find it helpful to have a mantra that works for me, such as, "I will help you when your body is calm." This allows me to give him minimal verbal support while letting him know that I will help him when he calms down but perhaps more important is that saying it reminds me to calm myself down.

Challenging Situation Map 1

I love mapping things out, so thinking about what challenging situations actually look like for me is really helpful. Knowing that my child is giving me feedback during these situations, as well as being mindful of the feedback that he is getting from me (or the adults who may be involved), also gives a lot of information to help everyone move forward in a more proactive and positive way.

If I were to map out the feedback flow chart I use, this is what it looks like for me...

Negative situation $\Longrightarrow$

Notice the feedback I'm being given $\Longrightarrow$

Pause and breathe $\Longrightarrow$

Zoom out and get curious - What is actually going on? What is my intention for this moment? ⟹

Zoom in and get curious. Based on what I'm noticing, what can I try to get back on track with my intention? ⟹

Use this feedback to try and see what might be helpful and if it isn't, go straight back to zooming in to try something different and see how that goes.

There is a good deal of experimenting involved but when I embrace my child archetype I can tap into curiosity aimed at supporting us. This leads to me noticing options I hadn't previously been aware of. This reduces frustration and also gives me insight into what works best for my child when he is experiencing challenging times.

Example:

Negative situation ⟹ *I'm annoyed because despite many reminders of when we are leaving for an appointment, my son is still in his room picking out the shirt he is going to wear.*

Notice the feedback I'm giving or being given ⟹ *He does not have the same sense of urgency that I have and insists on having more time to select his shirt. I'm starting to talk fast, sigh loudly and my tone/energy changes.*

Pause and breathe $\Longrightarrow$ *Self explanatory but very important!*

Zoom out and get curious - What is actually going on? What is my intention for this moment? $\Longrightarrow$ *What is actually going on is that I don't like being late and he needs to close the loop of getting dressed by picking out the shirt that he wants to wear. I also know that for him, there could be several things taking place, one being that he got distracted by electronics or something else in his room and the other being that making choices when there are a lot of options is challenging for him. Good to know AND remember!*

My intention for this moment is to calm myself, acknowledge that if we are a few minutes late, it will be okay.

Zoom in and get curious. Based on what I'm noticing, what can I try in order to get back on track with my intention? $\Longrightarrow$ *I can try to support him in any way that might help speed things up, offering to help narrow down his choices or play some sort of selection game (like "Eeny, meeny, miny, mo"). I can also get all of our stuff in the car, start the car, pull out of the garage so that when he comes out, we can leave right away. This all requires me to continue to take deep breaths, acknowledge that I'm annoyed but that he isn't doing it on purpose.*

Use this feedback to see what might work and if it doesn't, repeat in order to see if any other ideas you have might work. ⟹ After having these types of situations happen a few times, I realize that something has to change and this leads to conversations about strategies we can play with to see if they help us. Some that we've come up with for this particular situation are having him select his shirts for the week on Sunday by playing a dice game that his teacher helped him create. We also add 10-15 minute prep time before the actual time I would like to leave for where we are going. He does well with a timer so we have used that as well.

What typically happens in power struggles with a child? We get engrossed in the heat of the moment and do all we can do to put out the fires that are around us or feel like we are in a never-ending game of Whack A Mole. While this may result in a temporary fix for the moment, the arguing, yelling, bribing and manipulation that is typically involved in this sort of stop-gap strategy is an unnecessary drain on your emotional and physical energy - and rarely, if ever, leaves you feeling good.

Challenging Situation Description

Here is another description of how I zoom out during challenging times:

1. If I want to zoom out during a challenging time, the first thing I have to do is notice that something has shifted. I have to notice when a challenging type of situation is starting to happen, is happening, or has happened. This alone is a HUGE step in creating change!!! It is awesome because from there you can begin to be the observer and notice the thoughts you are having, the way your body feels and what emotions are coming up. This will help you to be more in tune with these so the next time it happens, you can do something different. Keep in mind though that like all of the other tools you've picked up along the way, it takes practice to build this new pattern.

2. Once you notice that you and your child have gone down an unhelpful path, mentally press pause for a second and take a deep breath.

3. Zoom out of the situation, almost like you are hovering above, looking down at a tv show set with characters acting out a scene.

4. From this perspective, get really curious. What do you notice in general? What do you notice about each of the characters (i.e.. Yourself, your child, your partner, the therapist or teacher, family members, etc.)?

What was happening before the situation led you down this path? Consider this question for every participant involved in the difficult episode. The wealth of information this provides can be very helpful in understanding the interactional dynamics that led to the episode, information that may allow you to avoid similar episodes in the future.

5. Notice your thoughts. Notice your emotions. Notice what you are feeling in your body.

Consider this example. You just have received an email from a teacher that made you mad and then you notice that your child is on their iPad again because they didn't know how to do their homework, didn't know what to do next or were bored. You snap at your child about how much they are on electronics and how you are going to take it from them which then sets them off and before you know it, you are in a heated battle of wills.

Or this scenario. You are happily making dinner in the kitchen and your child comes in from school, throws their stuff down and when you ask them nicely to pick it up, they go into a full blown meltdown, saying unkind things and possibly throwing things. From peace to chaos in 2.9 seconds.

Being an observer and getting curious can allow you to navigate these types of scenarios in very different ways because you can recognize what is actually going on, underneath the words or actions.

You will begin to notice your emotions and realize when you need to do something to process them.

You will begin to recognize how your child's emotions and energy are manifested differently depending on the challenges they've been confronting.

The information gained by zooming out is important and will help drive what is next.

6. Now zoom in. You've asked the question, "What is actually going on?" and have a better sense of what that might be.

From there, ask yourself, "What can I try right now to create a different result?" This question paired with utilizing the feedback that your child gives you about what works for them, what doesn't work for them, how they process information best, their learning style, etc. will make a huge difference!

Example:

Negative situation - One evening, my son became very upset because his dad ate a bite out of his chicken tender.

Feedback given - He slapped him on the shoulder to express this. My husband obviously didn't appreciate this and told him not to do that again. Words were exchanged and it wasn't fun.

Zoom out and get curious - When I zoomed out, I was able to see that this chicken tender was a leftover from a dinner he went to with his grandma. It was the only tender and he had saved it for dinner the next night.

What is our intention for this moment - To have a calm dinner experience.

Zoom in and get curious - Tell my husband what is actually going on and let him know that he would be angry if someone ate his only chicken tender and that an apology would be nice. I also had a conversation the next day with my son about how slapping is not okay and that there are other ways to express frustration, like saying, "Dude! It was not cool to take a bite of my chicken tender!"

Use feedback to see what could be done in the future - I didn't have to do anything. The next evening, when my husband came home, he apologized to our son and then without prompting, our son said, "I am going to offer you a bite of my tenders from now on so you don't have to just take them." Dad then said how much he appreciated this, we all moved on AND we were blown away at how he was able to come up with his own solution that was a compromise. So cool!!

Utilizing What You Know

We often have a treasure trove of information about our children that can go unnoticed or is forgotten. This is where bringing in your archetypes to team up and utilize what you know can make a world of difference. Here are some things that I personally like to consider. Does your child...

- do best with structures in place even if you don't like it or want to just go with the flow? (Schedules, timers, routines)
- do best with things written down (words or pictures), expressed verbally or actively engaged with? (Visual, auditory or kinesthetic learner)
- need downtime after experiences that might be challenging or overstimulating for them - academically, socially, emotionally, energetically? (School, therapy, extra-curricular activities, travel, parties, etc.)
- need food or drink frequently to keep them regulated?
- need less or more activities?
- need outlets for energy or ways to support their sensory system?
- need explicit directions?
- need support in doing things that might seem basic and like they "should" be able to do without?

The way you answer those questions can shift the situation from power struggle to one of curiosity with lots of options to get closer to desired outcome. The energy changes significantly and you may notice that your thoughts involve expectations that aren't reasonable in that moment.

This simple, yet powerful, ability to toggle between zooming in and zooming out is a game changer! Using it consistently will increase your confidence and competence to deal more efficiently and effectively with difficult situations.

Using the clarity building forces - curiosity, feedback and the three questions - personally allowed for a perspective that had playful energy as opposed to a rigid, controlling energy. I was able to let things go more easily knowing that next time, I could try different things. A bad day no longer left me feeling hopeless but rather gave me feedback about what I could try the next day to make it better.

Shifting from my "blinders on" approach to one filled with curiosity helped me look at my child through a different lens. I became more of an observer of him, noticing the different things that could impact his behavior, the underlying causes of behaviors, responses and strong emotions.

Learning to Untangle

Displays of strong emotional energy are like a vortex that can powerfully draw others into its trajectory. The ability to remain outside that vortex, keeping your own energy from becoming entangled in the chaos, is the ultimate practice in meditation...and very difficult to do. I often tell my clients that I would pay money to see how a Buddhist monk who meditates regularly would handle things with a child who is not regulated. It is easy to be clear and calm when alone or around others who are clear and calm and a whole other story when s#!t hits the fan with a child. In all seriousness, not getting tangled up requires awareness and acceptance of what is happening and the willingness to zoom out with curiosity.

Untangling from another person during times like this, especially when your child is involved, may seem counterintuitive. The strong empathic connection we have with our children predisposes us to move in closer when we witness our child in a state of distress or discomfort. But I have found that the ability to not get tangled up in what they are experiencing is generally the most effective way to help your child through these moments of heightened emotion. Untangling or not getting tangled up in the first place - physically, verbally, energetically - can help you to get perspective.

Margaret's Circles Tool

**This is one of my most helpful tools and is used in almost every coaching session I conduct.

It can be helpful to view your relationship with your child as a Venn Diagram - one circle being you and one circle being them, overlapping a bit. There are times when things are humming along nicely and your relationship might resemble a perfect Venn Diagram with a nice football shape in the middle.

There are also times when one person's energy is stronger and tries to dominate the other person. When that happens, the Venn Diagram changes and looks more like one circle covering the other up, which means there is little space for one person to think or communicate their thoughts or feelings. We can do this to our children and our children can do it to us. I can clearly remember doing this with very strong energy, trying to control my son's behavior which inevitably led to him responding by doing it right back to me with yelling, flopping, throwing, etc. This was one of the first "good to know" experiences I had with him that resulted in this visual/tool for me! What's perfect about that?!

When emotions get strong, the best thing I have found to do as a parent is to think about what I need to do in order to separate our circles, or scoot them over so the football shape in the center shrinks. This helps me to be able to breath, calm myself and get perspective on what might actually be going on with my child or myself.

If I can consciously minimize overlap or separate my energy from my son in those moments, I can be there for him in a much calmer, more supportive way. This not only helps me, but it helps him because I am not feeding into whatever is causing his distress or fueling the situation. My energy feels safe and steady and he can ride out the wave of his strong emotion at his own pace, which is generally much faster than if I've allowed myself to become entangled. And who doesn't want that?

If my son is upset and I get sucked into his strong emotion, I start having strong emotions and this never feels good. It also helps for me to remember that if I start getting upset with him, I am no longer in a position to best help him. This is not easy and is what I consider to be the ultimate in meditation - to be with someone who is experiencing strong feelings and not get sucked in and want to make it go away asap. So tough!!

When I am able to separate my circle from my son's circle during these times, I try to rewind the situation a bit to see if there is anything that stands out that could have triggered his strong emotional response.

I have found that a lot of people - including those who work with our children - often place the focus on the tantrum or the meltdown. They will tell you what the child did - they hit, they kicked, they yelled, they ran, they spit, they knocked things over, etc. But I find it much more effective and efficient to get curious about what was going on that led to the unexpected behavior or strong emotion, including asking myself what I may have done to contribute to the episode.

I remember getting calls and texts from my son's teacher about some unexpected behaviors and strong emotions in the classroom. The focus was on my son's behavior - the spitting, knocking things over and yelling - which usually led to him being taken to the office to calm down. She asked me why he was doing this and inquired about medication changes to "fix" this. Since I was not there and these explosions were uncharacteristic behaviors for him, it made me extremely curious about what was actually happening before he escalated so I could get a big picture perspective.

I wasn't there in the classroom and despite paying for a full time private aide for him, nobody was able to tell me what was going on other than that he was having strong emotional behaviors. As a former classroom teacher and educational consultant, this was quite confusing because something was causing these sudden escalations and medication wasn't the first thing I wanted to play around with.

One morning I got a glimpse of what was taking place and things started making complete sense to me.

Swinging was one of those activities that helped my son to regulate his body, which helped him transition into the school day. Allowing him some time to swing before school was part of a plan we (me and the school) came up with to support him. We would get to school early so that he could get on one of the two swings that were on the playground.

One day, we pulled into the driveway of the school, which happened to face the swings and as he got out, two boys pointed at my car and ran from where they were playing and jumped onto the swings. I saw my son come around the corner with a distressed look on his face. The boys had huge smiles on theirs. They knew exactly what they were doing...setting him up for a meltdown. Little did they know that they were messing with the wrong mom.

At the time, I was driving a convertible which looked a bit like a transformer when I would push the button to remove the roof. At that moment, I decided to see what would happen if I pushed the button. As the car started transforming from sedan to convertible, one of the boy's mouths dropped and he got off of the swing to get a closer look. As he did that, my son swooped in and got to swing. Ha! Take that suckers! (Not my most enlightened moment but I think if you are reading this, you'll understand how I felt.)

After that incident, I had a conversation with my son's team to let them know that this was probably not an uncommon thing and that they needed to keep an eye on those two boys when my son was around them. Turns out that things got much better and the explosive meltdowns lessened significantly. No medication changes necessary.

While not everything is going to be so obvious and clear as this example, your ability to "zoom out" will always prompt you to get curious. Getting curious can give you additional information about the underlying causes for your own child's behavior.

Once I have "zoomed out" to get the big picture view of the situation that is creating tension, I can begin to get clear on what I want and what actually matters in the moment (the "intention" part of the TIANT process). From there, I can then zoom in and play around with the "attention" part of

TIANT in order to ascertain what could have been done differently to achieve a more positive, satisfying outcome.

Approaching things this way has helped me to make changes that support us all in cycling through times like these so much faster.

Reminder - The TIANT Process stands for Tension, Intention, Attention and No (or Less) Tension.

After the Meltdown or Tantrum

Many of the tools I've introduced you to (noticing, curiosity, intention, questioning) can help you avert or reduce a meltdown or tantrum. Sometimes though, the meltdown will happen no matter what tools you've pulled out. When this happens, it is really important to allow emotions to get back to some sort of baseline once the meltdown or tantrum has ended. This doesn't mean that all is forgotten, it just means putting any conversations about what happened on hold.

What I find really helpful once we are back to that baseline energy is to reflect on the meltdown or tantrum in a manner that is aimed at supporting the child in finding alternative ways to manage things when they don't go as expected. I do this with a model that I've been using for years (introduced to me by his teacher Stacy Vinciguerra) that involves two rows of three circles.

The three circles represent (1) what led up to a response or reaction, (2) the response or reaction and (3) the outcome. The first row is what actually happened and the second row is where reflection and brainstorming can provide alternative responses or reactions and outcomes based on the same situation leading up to the response or reaction.

Example:

First row (what actually happened):

1. My son's iPhone wasn't plugged in to charge despite getting low battery messages and it died.
2. My son threw his iPhone on the ground.
3. I took the iPhone away, he tried to aggressively grab it back from me and the iPhone went into the safe.

Second row (the reflection and brainstorming):

1. My son's iPhone wasn't plugged in to charge despite getting low battery messages and it died.
2. Possible solutions - keep it plugged in while using it, ask for help when the low battery message appears, express disappointment and frustration using words or physically with something appropriate (hitting pillows or slamming a sandbag), make a plan to avoid this happening in the future, use a reminder, alarm or timer to remember to charge it, etc.

3. He gets to keep the iPhone and within a few minutes, the phone is ready to be used again while plugged in and charging.

In doing this sort of reflection process with him, I want to illustrate how different the results are between differing reactions and responses, and how trying to be more flexible and calm can help him to get back on track with what he's actually wanting.

I also have to be aware of the energy that I am bringing into any discussion around what happened. If I'm still upset or angry about it, chances are high that things are going to escalate again. This is where being aware of thoughts, emotions and how the body responds to challenging situations can be really helpful. I might think I'm "fine" but my tone and energy, including my needs for what he "should" do or say, are going to be evident to him.

When I seek to understand the dynamics of my son's meltdowns from a place of pure curiosity, I often find that my thoughts and emotions are less about punishment and consequences or needing him to do or say anything, but rather are focused on what I can do to support his learning and growth. And frequently, doing this has helped me realize that I'm expecting behaviors that are outside his developmental range.

From there I can better deflect any defensiveness. realize that there might be some embarrassment, confusion, anxiety, feelings of being wronged or not in control, etc. on his part and that will help me engage him in a supportive conversation to explore together what actually happened and how a similar scenario could be addressed in the future.

Consequences

When a child has a tantrum or meltdown, it typically leads to the discussion of consequences (or "outcomes" based on the 3 circle method just introduced). This can be a tricky topic to dive into, especially if your child is on their own developmental timeline. First, let's get clear on what we mean by consequences. For the purposes of this chapter, consequences can be either natural or imposed, and are meant to reinforce a desired behavior.

Natural consequences are related to the result of an action-touch a hot stove and you get burned. Imposed consequences are chosen by someone else. Since this is a book about parenting, l want to focus mostly on consequences chosen by parents for their child, particularly in times of stress, which was something I had a hard time with.

Because we cannot control how or if our children are able to interpret the consequences of their actions, it is vital to remember what we know about our child and use that to guide how we support them in order to learn and grow. A child may not want to or be able to assign meaning to a consequence - natural or imposed. This may seem surprising to some, however a lot of parents on the hero's journey in parenting struggle with the fact that their children, like mine, could care less about losing something unless it is meaningful to them and/or they aren't able to make the connection between their response or reaction and the outcome.

> This is why I like the 3 circle method as it not only creates a visual of this, it also allows you to be specific with them about alternate responses or reactions and see more positive outcomes.

With regards to imposed consequences as it applies to parenting, the first step is to get clear on what your intention is for the consequence because if you are not clear on exactly what you want to occur and why you want it, you will react based on what you feel you "should" do or what your personal experiences have been.

When you choose to impose a consequence on your child, it also needs to be appropriate for your child's developmental stage. After all, if a toddler reaches out towards a hot stove - you don't explain how heat speeds up molecular activity and causes tissue damage - you just grab their hand and move it, sometimes with an associated keyword "Hot!". Similarly, you don't put them in time out or take away their favorite toy for the rest of the day. Remembering to use what you know about what works and what doesn't work for you and your child during times like this can also make a big difference.

Over the years I have noticed a few different patterns that create confusion during tension filled times.

- In the heat of the moment people throw out consequences as an attempt to get a meltdown or tantrum to stop. (Been there, done that!) A lot of times those consequences are more than what the situation requires OR are more than what is appropriate for the child, such as "If you don't stop right now, you will lose electronics for the rest of your life!", especially when you consider the underlying cause of the meltdown or tantrum.

- A parent will avoid imposing a consequence due to fear of the child's reaction/response to them. "If I make my child clean up the mess they made, they are just going to yell and make more of a mess."

Again, consequences are a natural part of everyone's lives and when it comes to parenting, every family needs to decide for themselves how they want to use consequences to address problem behaviors based on what works best for your child as well as the challenges that your family faces.

If you do choose to impose a consequence, I recommend taking a momentary pause to consider what is reasonable, doable and obtainable for the child, given your intention for the consequence.

I use "If...then..." statements with my son - "If you plug your phone or iPad in when you are not using it, then it will be charged." This way he understands that if he chooses to do or not do something, then that choice has a positive or negative consequence.

If you are worried that setting a consequence will inflame the current situation, pressing the pause button and getting curious might be appropriate. Perhaps the child is embarrassed and ashamed by what they did. Adding a consequence to those intense feelings would likely intensify them. In that situation, working to help them find a way to make amends could be a meaningful lesson.

They may also feel that what they did was an appropriate response to some sort of "wrong-doing" that they felt they experienced. Perhaps your child dumped a playmate's crayon box on the floor after his friend made fun of the picture your son was drawing. With as little verbal engagement as possible, work with them, possibly assigning them 2 or 3 things to be in charge of picking up. If that doesn't work, I would at least have them stay in the area until things have been put back together.

I have also learned to get curious about what sort of consequence is actually needed in order to support my intention. Many times a five minute electronics break has the same impact as losing it for an hour or a day. Him calming his body and being able to earn it back helps us all get back to baseline much faster.

I think it is important to be mindful of the energy that is going into interactions around consequences. Finding a balance of what feels supportive and empathetic without providing a shadow payoff for strong emotional responses to the situation seems to work best for us.

> Co-regulation when a child is dysregulated is totally different
> from providing a shadow payoff.

An example of a shadow payoff for something like the phone or iPad dying could be me giving him a big hug right after he throws the device on the ground because it died.

I definitely want to support him not allowing the device to die and I want to acknowledge that I know it's frustrating when it does. But giving him a hug as a way of empathizing with his situation sends a mixed message. It's as if I'm telling him, "It's irresponsible to let your device die when we've provided you with many cords and charging stations for that purpose. And it's definitely unacceptable to throw an expensive phone on the floor and possibly break it - but I'll be affectionate when you do that.

My intention is to not get tangled up in the frustration that he may be experiencing with himself for not charging his device despite the reminders of low battery. I want to support him in what this experience has taught him and what could be done differently the next time so he doesn't have to become frustrated and angry with his device. Once we've gone through this, I am MORE than happy to give him all the hugs he wants.

If possible, I like to focus on the "What's perfect about this?" question surrounding what this natural consequence has helped us to learn, practice or remember. Putting our Storyteller to work in finding those things can help to shift the energy from negative to positive. If he cannot think of anything, I can offer up what I notice or what it would have taught me in order to start building this new muscle for him. (This is why it is important for me to play with this and intentionally point out my own "What's perfect about this?" lessons around my own natural consequences...so he knows it's not just him.)

If he is not ready to learn from the consequences, that is alright. I know that there are times I'm not ready, so I cannot expect him to be any different. As a parent, I want to model that there is a choice around how we eventually look at something that can create a feeling of empowerment as opposed to staying in a victim mentality.

Your Child IS Learning from You!

I knew my son understood the concept of consequences when he composed a letter to me and my husband. (He does things like this with me all of the time!) He does not like flies in the house (who does?), but it really bothers him. We have three dogs who need to go outside and sometimes flies will come in when the door is opened to let them out or back in. He gets very upset about this. When he was 16 years old, he composed a letter that he taped on the window of the door. I cannot find the original but it was something like...

"To avoid the consequences of letting flies in, the door cannot be open for more than 3 seconds."

This totally cracked me up and let me know that he understands that a person can have wants as part of a family. It also told me he understood that other members of the family can impact those wants. Not sure what the consequences were going to be, probably scotch taping the door shut, but he was clear that there would be some if what he wanted didn't happen. Great lesson in seeing how we are all interconnected in family relationships!

Reset Button/Do Over

If you find yourself feeling strong emotions and either throwing out unrealistic consequences or avoiding them altogether, you are not alone! I've often had to press the "reset" button on either an unrealistic consequence I set for my son or didn't set when one would have been helpful. Acknowledging this allowed me to get back on track by shifting back to something that WAS realistic or finding a way to communicate to him that what happened didn't feel great and that if there was a next time like this, I was going to have a different response.

> In either of these cases, I do try to engage him in being part of the process in determining what would be appropriate. This helps me to provide support for my child while also being clear about the lesson behind the consequence's intention. Also, if in lieu of a consequence to some intentional misbehavior I tell my son to expect a different response the next time it happens, it is critical that I follow

> through with that expectation. It is ill-advised to threaten a consequence that you are unwilling to impose.

Pressing the "reset" button or having a "Do-Over" can be helpful if the child is open to it. This tool works especially well if embarrassment is the source. A "Do-Over" means taking a deep breath and letting go of whatever has happened and re-doing it in a more positive way than what was happening before the meltdown or tantrum.

Example:

One Friday evening, my mother-in-law and my grandmother-in-law (92 years old) were over for pizza and my son had been working with his occupational therapist on eating pizza (a sensory challenge for him). I cut a sliver of pizza and put it on his plate. I thought nothing of it and we all sat at the counter eating our food until he noticed it and said, "WTF is this pizza doing on my plate?" (There were actual words used, not initials!)

Eyebrows were raised and the eyes of my in-laws got huge as you can imagine. My initial response was thinking I should get big with my energy in order to show these women that I respect, that this was not okay. Then I remembered what I know, which is that getting big with my energy with my son does not work. Ever. It only escalates things.

I walked over to him and took the phone that he was playing Minecraft on. He grabbed it back and I looked at him and calmly said, "You can either give me your phone and get it back today or I will take it and you will not get it back until tomorrow." He handed it to me and I went into my bedroom to sit and calm myself down.

He came in and sat in the chair next to me. I was taking deep breaths and after about 10 seconds he said, "Can I have a do-over?" I asked, "What would the do-over look like?" He said, "I will try the pizza and not yell and will lose electronics for 15 minutes." I added, "And you will apologize to your grandma and great grandma for using strong language in front of them."

He did this all and we were back to baseline in less than 5 minutes. Personally, I would have accepted this all without losing electronics but hey, it was his idea!

Chapter Twenty-Three

Looking Inward During the Stormy Times of Parenting

Noticing what might be going on within you during stormy times that are frustrating, intense and challenging is extremely important. While it was super humbling for me to become aware of the thoughts and energy I was bringing to those situations, it also empowered me because I realized I could do things differently only when I began to notice what was not working. Doing things differently always ended up making a difference for both of us in positive ways.

Here are some questions I would ask myself:

- *Am I trying to control my child or the situation? Do I have internal rules about what "should" be happening or how my child "should" be?*
- *Am I doing too many things at once? (I noticed that quite often I was in my head thinking about a situation while I was preparing a meal or cleaning*

*something up. I would then react in a negative
way when there was any other need/want that
came onto my radar.)*

- *Am I engaging in verbal or energetic battles with
  my child? Are they pushing my "trigger buttons"
  in order to get me to engage?*
- *Am I falling back into old, learned, familiar patterns that I know do not work for us?*
- *Am I needing self care in some form, even if it is a
  minute in the bathroom to take some deep breaths
  and regroup?*
- *Am I being curious about what actually might be
  the underlying cause of my child's strong emotions
  or behaviors OR am I just ignoring those causes
  with the hope that it will all go away?*

These questions do NOT imply judgment of any kind! When
I can be curious and open about my answers, I am better able
to press pause and get back on track with what I know works
for my son. If I do not get curious, nothing changes...which
is good to know!!

Once I have an idea of what might be going on, I can utilize
tools to help us get back on track. There are two very helpful
things for me to remember during these times. The first is
checking in with my intention for the moment, which might
be different from what it was two minutes earlier, and, second,
doing what I can to help us reset and get back to baseline.

And, of course, it almost always helps to get curious about what actually matters and what I can do to support my child.

Example:

While I am writing this, we are on a ski trip and I have learned that when we go skiing, there are a lot of Executive Functioning skills necessary for him to employ in getting himself ready and if there is additional pressure, he will either escalate or shut down. His usual morning routine involves eating breakfast, taking care of his hygiene stuff, getting dressed, and making the bed.

Our morning routine is very similar when we go skiing. However, getting dressed is a much more challenging task. There are many layers that need to go on in a certain order. The layers are often snug and not easy to get on. I used to do it all for him, laying clothing out in order, helping him get it all on. But, as he has gotten older and more independent with it, I have limited my help to the outer layers and boots.

We do what we can to give him time to do all of these things in order to be ready for his adaptive ski lesson on time and he has a "Reminders" list of what is needed in the order that works best.

This morning he did almost everything on his own (boots are still tough) and was right on schedule to leave for his lesson. YAY!! He left and I walked past his room with his bed unmade and thought, "What actually matters right now? Does it matter that his bed is unmade?" No! What mattered this morning was that he got ready on his own and was on time!

I took a few moments to make his bed because I wanted to do that for him. Will I make his bed when we get back home? Nope. Here, sure, because I want him to focus on other things that don't come as easily to him and have evidence that doing so over and over again has helped him to be more independent and feel more competent.

Executive functioning challenges often require a lot of deep breaths from us as parents because things that may seem simple to us or things that we have explained or they have done a million times might still feel like it is the first time they are doing something. Accepting and acknowledging that this is where they are at this moment can help reduce thoughts like "They should know how to do this by now!" or "I shouldn't have to tell them this every single day." Acknowledging that this is what is needed for them RIGHT NOW can reduce feelings of frustration. If the intention is for them to be able to complete some task, and the process toward achieving that goal requires breaking it down into shorter, doable parts and pieces, then that is where your supportive attention can be directed.

Margaret-ism
Awareness of Trigger Buttons

"Trigger buttons" are those things that can set you off, bother you, irritate you, etc. and they are unique to each person. Our children are especially good at identifying our trigger buttons and, under certain circumstances, they have no qualms about pushing those buttons to try to engage us, typically in a negative way.

For example, my son figured out that I didn't like it when things were slammed or when furniture was tipped over. Knowing this, when he was upset and I wasn't engaging the way he wanted, he would tip over the kitchen chairs. He even slammed the oven door down a few days before Thanksgiving and broke the door's spring. This meant our oven wouldn't close and wouldn't heat up without duct taping the door therefore we roasted and baked our dinner with tape holding the door closed that year!

My son figured out his dad's trigger button and when they would get into disagreements, he would do all he could to push it. Both of these were not obvious to us until I noticed the pattern that he was presenting us with - "If I do this, then they respond this way." (Here are consequences again!)

Being aware of our trigger buttons, as well as the fact that he knew how to push them, allowed us to anticipate his button pushing behavior with calmer energy and more thoughtful responses. Fairly quickly, he stopped doing them. He absolutely tries new things all of the time, however, we know that they are just attempts to push our trigger buttons and we try not to respond with strong energy because we know what is actually going on.

The next time that you are experiencing a challenging time with your child, get curious about how they are trying to engage you. Are they doing something they know drives you crazy? This might give you some insight into your own personal trigger buttons.

> Since everyone has them, learning to recognize your child's trigger buttons can help you better support them in peer or sibling relationships or in school or sporting activities.

Part Five Conclusion: Summary, Key Concepts and Power Questions

Summary:

Becoming more familiar with how Hindering Forces show up in your life as a parent can help you to feel more prepared to support yourself and your child. You can also be more prepared to use what you know in order to be more effective and efficient with the energy you are putting into countering those forces.

This feels so much better than feeling like they sneak up on you, coming out of nowhere. Chances are there are patterns and using skills like noticing, curiosity, intention and questioning can offer you the ability to recognize what is actually going on, as opposed to battling behaviors that are the result of Hindering Forces, and help you get back on track faster.

Key Concepts:

- Common Causes of Meltdowns and Tantrums:
  1. Sensory Overload
  2. Emotional Regulation Challenges
  3. Embarrassment

4. Chronological Age vs Development Age
5. Learning Stage Exhaustion
6. Desire to Control and Testing Boundaries
7. The Need to Close an Open Loop

- *For PDA, check out Dr. Melissa Neff and for Executive Functioning Challenges, check out Seth Perler. Both have done podcasts with Debbie Reber on TiLT Parenting.
- Venn Diagram Circles Tool
- Reset Button/Do Over
- Trigger Buttons

Power Questions:

- Is there something I can do in advance to support my child during typical times of sensory overload?
- If strong emotions or an inability to regulate emotions is like a fire, what can I do in order to support my child while also not adding fuel to the fire?
- If there is a strong response or reaction to something going wrong or not as expected, could your child be embarrassed?
- How old is my child developmentally right now?
- How much time is my child spending a day in the different learning stages?
- What are some unconsciously competent activities that my child enjoys?

- Is my child trying to get me to engage in a power struggle? If so, why do I think they are doing so? Are they getting a shadow payoff?
- Is my child upset because there is an open loop that they need/want to be closed? If so, what are some ways I can play around with to close the loop even if just temporarily?
- What is actually going on right now?
- What actually matters in this moment?
- What do I know about my child?
- What is going on within me during challenging times?
- What are my trigger buttons?

PART SIX

Empowering Forces

Up to this point I have introduced you to shadow aspects of the Warrior, the Storyteller, the Battle Ready Bodyguard, the Guardian of Your Heart, as well as Hindering Forces like control and judgment. If you are anything like me, you most likely have encountered at least one or two of these along the way on your hero's journey in parenting. I have shared some tools to help empower and support yourself by shifting your relationship with those forces. I now want to highlight a number of Empowering Forces that you always have access to that can support you every step of the way.

- Empowering Force #1: Creating Balanced Flow
- Empowering Force #2: Self Care

- Empowering Force #3: Gratitude
- Empowering Force #4: Intentional Parenting Using Archetypes
- Empowering Force #5: Actively Seeking and Creating Joy
- Empowering Force #6: Setting Myself Up for Success

You may remember way back at the beginning of this book where I shared how there was little joy in my life, especially in parenting. That powerful awareness nudged me to answer the call to this hero's journey and the wild unknown adventure of parenting my child. You may also be wondering why we didn't just jump into this part of the journey right away as surely it would be more fun, right?!

I get it! I wanted that as well. However, I learned that I couldn't simply leap frog over the tools, questions and strategies shared previously because they were necessary in order to get me to the point where I could allow myself to truly feel joy.

I intentionally held off shining a light on these until later on in this book because I know the incredible power these Shadow and Hindering Forces can have. They can be extremely convincing as they persuade you to stay right where you are, often leading you to feeling uncertain, inadequate and alone, all under the guise of keeping you safe. You now have ways to approach them with empowered awareness, knowing that there is so much more connection to yourself and your child when you are able to be open and curious.

I had to first learn that the thoughts my Storyteller was creating weren't always true. I had to relax my Battle Ready Bodyguard so that I could reconnect to my body and notice what the tension was trying to tell me. I had to reassure the Guardian of My Heart that all would be okay if I released years of stored emotion and felt the pure emotions in safe and healthy ways. I needed to build a new relationship with all of these things in order to be able to be connected with my authentic self so I could empower myself against control and judgment. Once I connected to my authentic self, I could once again feel joy.

Just to refresh your memory, here are some of the tools covered so far...

- TIANT Process (Tension, Intention, Attention, No (or less) Tension
- The Storyteller - Listening to their "stories" with greater discernment
- Demoting the Battle Ready Bodyguard
- Creating a new relationship with the Guardian of Your Heart
- The Power of Stillness
- Byron Katie's Inquiry Process (Four Questions)
- Awareness of Judgment and Not Handing Over Power
- Curiosity
- Control vs. Influence

Chapter Twenty-Four

Empowering Force #1 - Creating a More Balanced Flow of Energy

Creating a more balanced flow of energy in parenting (and in life) requires both "doing" and "being." Most parents on the hero's journey in parenting find themselves primarily in "doing" mode without any "being" activities and if so, they typically get boomerang-ed right back into "doing" mode. Over time, this leads to exhaustion and judgment.

This is how I operated for the first seven years of my son's life. I tried so many different things and was doing x, y and z to try and manage each situation. I didn't spend any time celebrating even the smallest of things that went well. I also didn't spend any time reflecting on what worked. This meant I wasn't integrating what was learned into the next experience and as a result, I was constantly reinventing the wheel.

Once I realized that this was happening, I began to look more intentionally at the cycle of "doing" and "being" energies that make up the natural energy cycle I referenced earlier from

"Coyote's Guide to Connecting with Nature" by Ellen Haas, Evan McGown and Jon Young. This helped me gain a fresh understanding of how each direction and its energy is necessary in order to support me in parenting.

When I began to be more intentional about going through each energy, even if only in the tiniest ways, things really started to flow in a more balanced and empowering manner with my son. This felt wonderful and I want the same for you!

As I used the natural energy cycle more and more, I also began to notice that if I skipped or omitted a part of the cycle, I felt "off" but couldn't put my finger on why. Having a framework of the different natural energies and the importance of them in this cycle was important in helping me during those "off" times to get back on track.

To refresh your memory, the directions and their energies of this cycle are...

NE - Intention

E - Inspiration

SE - Preparation

S - Action

SW - Relaxation and Recovery

W - Celebration

NW - Reflection

N - Integration

Example:

(NE) Intention: To leave the house with my son feeling calm and prepared for wherever we are going.

Intention is a wonderful place to start and allows your Monarch/Elder archetype to get clarity around what you are wanting and why you are wanting it. *(This is the "I" part of my TIANT Process.)* When tension rises and things go awry, intention can be brought in (or back in) by pressing pause and getting still, even if just for a few seconds. Intention can reconnect you with what actually matters in the present moment.

(E) Inspiration: We've been able to leave the house to go on playdates or to the pool feeling calm in the past, so I know it is possible!

Inspiration is the place of curiosity and play! It can guide you in better understanding what sort of *attention* could be given to support your intention. Inspiration can come from many different sources such as other people, a story, a memory, etc. Inspiration is a pivotal part of the desire to create change.

**(The rest are all aspects of the "A" part of my TIANT Process.)

(SE) Preparation: I am going to sit down, possibly with a sheet of paper, and map out what is actually needed in order to make this happen. In this part of the energy cycle, I'm thinking about all of the parts and pieces. I'm thinking about where we are going and what we are doing so I can use my Storyteller in a productive way. I can also tell myself "This is doable!" instead of telling myself "This is going to be a disaster."

Preparation is just what it sounds like...the prepping and planning needed in order to support yourself and your child in doing what you can to move closer towards your intention.

(S) Action: Once I have my mental or written out map, I can start taking action on the specific details of what is actually needed to accomplish my intention. For this particular example, I can get out my tote bag and start loading it with anything we might need.

If mornings are typically rushed and stressful —as they are for many parents— I would recommend doing what you can the evening before to prepare. For example, I will try to find a place in the refrigerator to batch the items that I want to bring. Or I may fill a lunch box with snack items and set it on the counter in an obvious location. Any paperwork needed for doctor or therapy appointments is printed and put in the tote bag so it is done and not forgotten.

It may seem too obvious to say that achieving a desired outcome requires some sort of action on our part. Of course it does! But part of the beauty and power of the natural energy cycle comes from how it turns general, nonspecific action into meaningful action.

In fact, the ACTION phase of the energy cycle could more accurately be called Targeted or Informed Action to highlight the fact that it flows naturally from knowing precisely the "what" and "why" of our intended outcome (INTENTION), is energized by the motivational impetus of INSPIRATION, and is guided by PREPARATION of a specific plan.

Utilizing this foundation, we can now proceed toward our intended outcome with more confidence and a clearer understanding of the behavioral steps necessary to get there, especially those first small steps that are often the most difficult to take in order to get the snowball of change rolling downhill.

Tips:

- If you tend to forget things that you had intended on bringing, make yourself a note or list to leave on the counter or in the driver's seat to check before leaving.

(SW) Rest/Recovery: This can happen either once I get into the car (even just for a second), once we get to wherever we are going or when we return home. Oftentimes it involves taking a deep breath and allowing myself to simply enjoy that we made it out of the house without sweating.

Relaxation and Recovery is important because it is draining to be in action mode - physically, mentally, and emotionally. This often feels uncomfortable because the Storyteller and Battle Ready Bodyguard create thoughts and bodily tension around why you "shouldn't" do this (common stories involve there being too much to do, not enough time, and laziness).

> If you do allow for stillness, it often creates fertile ground for new ideas or approaches that feel urgent to act on, sending you right back into action mode with a new intention without celebration, reflection and integration. Bypassing these and springing right back into action mode is what I call the boomerang effect and keeps you from all of the benefits of the rest of the cycle's energies.

Having connection with some form of awareness building so that you can notice when those aspects of the Warrior archetype, the Shadow Forces, take over is extremely helpful. Noticing the tension that occurs when this happens and having the ability to realize what is actually going on in the moment can allow you to take a deep breath, thank your archetypes for trying to help you, albeit in a misguided way, and give yourself permission to give your body and mind what it is needing to refuel.

This is self care and I will expand on this in the next section, but for now, it could include things like stillness, taking a nap, lying on a hammock, watching a favorite show, taking a bath, going for a leisurely walk, etc. It is essentially finding a way to slow down and just "be" in the moment without exerting a lot of energy.

> This also doesn't have to be a long period of time or done alone because, of course, I am realistic that we have real lives and children that cannot be ignored.

(W) Celebration: I allow myself to celebrate the smallest of wins, even if things didn't go perfectly. One piece of the process going well is worth celebrating! My son might struggle or forget something AND I can still appreciate the impact I've made by preparing the night before.

I'm convinced that celebrations happen too rarely in parenting our children. Celebrating our successes, both large and small, helps keep us moving confidently forward by infusing our attitude, energy and emotion with passion and conviction. Acknowledging anything that supports you and/or your child in learning and growing deserves to be celebrated.

Allow yourself to feel the good feelings - contentment, joy, love, awe, pride, gratitude - even when they may be fleeting. I will often hear from clients about small gains that they have in parenting or something that their child has done and there is usually a "but" inserted immediately afterwards as though it wasn't big enough to actually be celebrated. This usually leads me to interrupt and proclaim, "Do you realize that this is so awesome and HUGE!?!" The typical response is something like, "You're right! It actually is a big thing."

Allow yourself to feel the good feelings!

(NW) Reflection: Celebration ties in nicely with reflection. Oftentimes we don't take the time to reflect on things; however, when we do allow ourselves the time to zoom out and see things from a different perspective, we realize that even the tough spots we've lived through (maybe especially the tough spots) contain nuggets of learning and growth that can make the next tough spot less stressful. That's a big deal!!

Reflection can involve taking a few moments to journal or revisit those questions I shared earlier - What worked? What didn't work? What is one thing that could be done differently the next time? I love cycling through those questions because they help me focus my attention in an effective and efficient manner and help me focus less on any thoughts or judgments that may have popped up based on what happened. I can then share what I've learned from considering these questions with my husband and my son to help ensure that we are approaching things together from a realistic perspective, and not some idealistic vision that is unattainable

Creating awareness through reflection also means that you are creating new pathways in your brain that make it easier in real time to distinguish helpful patterns and tendencies from unhelpful ones. This is extremely empowering.

An example of my reflection process for this particular situation is to think about whether or not we had everything we needed/wanted to make our outing as successful and enjoyable as it could be. Did we have enough time or were we feeling rushed? If everything was going smoothly, was I able to relax and actually feel calm or did I revert to feeling stressed because that is how I normally feel?

If something worked, awesome! Take note of that so that I can remember to try that again the next time. If something didn't work, awesome! Without judgment or shaming, what was it and what did it teach me? Now I have more information, so I can try something different the next time.

(N) Integration: Based on what I learned during the experience, how do I want to integrate that learning into future experiences? Is there anything I need or want to do in order to set myself or my child up for success? What can I/we do to influence a more positive outcome?

I know that I do best when I take a few minutes to think through what my son and I are probably going to want or need. I never used to do this, relying solely on my ability to go with the flow and put out fires as they flared up. While I can still choose to do this, it never feels good. Plus I never really feel the ease and joy that I desire.

My son does best when he has enough time and isn't feeling rushed. Knowing this, I always try to create a false leave time. This way, we have a buffer in case he gets distracted or something takes longer than expected. He also does well when he knows what he needs to do beforehand, preferably in writing. So I text him or print out a checklist, which he likes and requests, so he can process it visually as opposed to me telling him.

Integration is all about taking what you have learned throughout this cycle into other situations in order to better support you and your child. Not doing this reminds me of the popular saying about how doing the same thing over and over again and expecting a different result is the definition of insanity. Making a plan for implementing a small shift or change based on what you have learned about yourself and/or your child is helpful and eventually creates a snowball effect with more and more to celebrate.

As I continuously went through this cycle, I felt more empowered even if things didn't go as planned. I was less vulnerable to the results because I knew that there was always something new for me to learn. Sure there have been many times when I want to put the white flag up and say, "Enough learning opportunities for now please!!" But even when times feel overwhelming, the awareness and intentionality of this cycle helps me to feel capable of creating changes that feel better for us all.

Importantly, and perhaps surprisingly, using the energy cycle to better balance my energy flow has improved my ability to communicate more effectively to others the things that are either supporting or undermining my intention. An obvious example is how much easier it has become to share with my son when changes need to be made and why they are being made. I'm confident this positive change can be attributed to the clarity that comes with giving myself more time in "being energy" rather than spending all my energy on "doing".

Using the Natural Balance of Energy Cycle with Doctors, Therapists or Professionals

Intention: My intention is to discuss areas of tension or concern with a professional in order to get information or ideas around how to better support my child.

Inspiration: Tapping into curiosity in order to approach supporting my child in any way possible. Perhaps this appointment came as a result of a recommendation of a trusted friend, or from a concern that I have about my child and their development.

Preparation: I used to just go into appointments and meetings like these assuming that I was the novice, and they were the experts who would be able to give me the answers I needed. Since those early days of handing my power over to them, I have learned that it is important for me to check in with my intention and jot down questions or curiosities that I have before the appointment. This way I can have them ready to bring up and not rely on the assumption that they are going to know what I want or need in order to support my son.

I also recognize that meetings or appointments like this can be extremely stressful and intimidating, so doing what I can to make myself feel comfortable and confident is important. For me this means wearing clothes that make me feel comfortable and confident as well as reminding myself that at the "every day" experiential level I know my child better than they do.

Action: Bringing a list of questions or concerns to these appointments helps keep me from being overwhelmed by new information and reduces the anxiety that comes from having to rely on my memory. Doing things that help me be clear about my intention, like remembering that I'm there to gather information and that I'm not required to make any decision at that moment, ensures that the ACTION phase doesn't turn into a REACTION phase.

Self Care/Recovery: After the appointment or meeting, I take some time, even if it is just a few minutes to breathe in order to care for myself knowing that what I just did was probably tough and perhaps heard some things about my child that require processing because maybe they stung, even if they were confirming a hunch.

This may also include running through the Starbucks drive-thru to get a favorite coffee or taking a nap once home or getting take-out for dinner rather than cooking. There are many little ways to care for yourself in order to refuel after a challenging time.

Celebration: Just as important as self care and recovery, it is a good thing to allow myself even just a moment to acknowledge and celebrate how I was able to get through a tough meeting or conversation. Celebration can tag along with a self care strategy. It could involve an intentional, metaphorical hug, high five or calling a friend!!

Reflection: Reflecting on a meeting or appointment in order to learn from and get clarity around what was discussed can be extremely helpful. Use the following questions to help you reflect:

- What did I learn?
- What do I need to learn more about?
- What felt true or in alignment with my child and/or our family?
- What didn't feel true or in alignment with my child or our family?
- What questions do I still have?
- What do I need some clarity around in order to make a decision?

Integration: I can use the information that I gathered during the meeting or appointment to make decisions and choices to help us all move forward. This can involve adding or subtracting things from our routine. It means knowing when to say "yes" or "no" to things. Having additional conversations or information gathering sessions in order to further understand how to support my child and our family is also an excellent way to integrate and reinforce previously learned information.

Utilizing the natural energy cycle has helped me tremendously by checking in on what directional energies I am utilizing most for support and which ones I may be underutilizing. The more that I do this, the more it helps to set me up to successfully help my future self out. Something we will dive into in the next chapter!

Chapter Twenty-Five

Empowering Force #2 - Setting Myself Up for Success

Setting myself up for success is an Empowering Force that doesn't come naturally to me. I am really good, talented, if I may say so myself, at making things more difficult than they need to be and then feeling stressed out. This self-handicapping strategy and its consequences cause a tremendous amount of tension in my life. Shocking, right?! However, as I began to play with being more intentional in how I wanted to feel, I noticed that what I wanted most of all was to feel ease and joy.

Once I recognized that those were the feeling states that I was trying to have more of in my life, I began to utilize my TIANT Process more and more by recognizing what was causing tension, getting clarity around my intention, being curious about what attention could support my intention so that I could have no (or less) tension.

This helped me gain a keen awareness of what was keeping me from having what I was wanting - ease and joy - and from there, I could try different ways of doing things in order to influence and increase the possibility that these feeling states could come to fruition.

My tendency has always been to jump right into things, work hard, feel busy and "pinball" through my day. Because this doesn't always work out so great and creates opposite feeling states from what I desire, I have had to learn to notice this and then press pause.

Noticing is the key to awareness and pressing pause helps me remember and reconnects me with my intention. From there I can redirect my energy and attention so that I can support that intention.

So what does this look like in parenting? Let's consider a relatively common occurrence at our house — taking my son to the pool. My desire always is to do this with as much ease and joy as possible. However, nine times out of ten something gets forgotten which causes a great deal of tension between us. Knowing this is a pattern, something had to change if I wanted less tension.

This sounds basic, but this was not something that came naturally to me. I had to recognize the tension that was created by the three Shadow Forces -

1. My Storyteller would tell me all sorts of stories filled with "shoulds" directed at me and my son. (He *should* remember that he needs his goggles. I *should* remember to check the bag before we leave

the house. We *should* just stay home.)

2. The Guardian of the Heart was trying to protect me from feelings of frustration, annoyance and despair but since I'm feeling them already, they seep out into the interactions I have with my son. (Ugh! I just want to scream and cry! Why does this always have to be so hard? I just wanted a fun and relaxing outing with him. I don't want to have to go back home to get the goggles but if I don't, he's not going to swim which defeats the purpose of going to the pool.)

3. My Battle Ready Bodyguard would create lots of tightness throughout my body as it tried to defend me from the feelings associated with the stories. (Stomach tightens as it prepares for a punch in the gut resulting from his anxiety and disappointment. My jaw clenched in frustration with myself and wanting to yell because we have been here before and we both *should* know better.)

> All of this happens in a split second and I'm sure you can think of examples where this has played out for you with your child.

When it happens, I know this is not how I want to feel so I have to take a minute and think about what I can do to change the pattern and create ease and joy in situations like this.

A favorite question I use...

What can I do to help my future self out?

...allow my Storyteller to use what it knows to envision what it could look like to support my future self. Storytellers are brilliantly skilled at coming up with narratives regarding some less than successful event or outing---and usually in a way that presents me in a less than favorable light. But by actively recruiting my Storyteller to brainstorm possible strategies that can help support me IN THE FUTURE, I'm allowing my Storyteller to work FOR me.

After asking this question about the pool situation I described above, we now have a pool bag that lives in the laundry room which is by the garage door. It contains all that we need, sunscreen, flip flops, swimsuit, towels and even an extra pair of goggles for "just in case" situations. This makes it easy because everything is in one place and I just have to grab it and go.

It lives in the laundry room so that when the swimsuits and towels are dry, they go right into the bag which means they don't get lost in my son's bedroom. It also contains a printed list of items that need to be in there so we can check and make sure it's all there before leaving the house.

> Using something like a luggage tag with a bulleted list inside the plastic cover and attaching it to the bag's handle so it is readily available helps to make it super easy to do a quick check before heading out. This could also be placed on a backpack as well to encourage going through

a checklist before leaving for school and also before leaving school at the end of the day.

Asking the question "What can I do to help my future self out?" never fails me. It often encourages me to do things that maybe I don't really want to do at the moment, like getting gas when I still have a quarter tank left or unloading the dishwasher, but I know that my future self will be grateful and I'm always happy that I've created more ease and joy for myself by taking the five minutes to do those things.

Tending to my future self in this way empowers me to get out in front of the endless tension-producing scenarios that pop up unexpectedly time and time again. It also works hand in hand with the three questions I shared earlier:

- What works?
- What doesn't work?
- What is something I can do differently the next time to get a more positive result?

Taking a little bit of time to consider these questions around an area of tension helps me use what I know rather than disregard all of the valuable information that I have at my disposal from past experiences...good and bad.

The following are common situations that come to mind when helping one's future self.

Leaving the House

I like to gather or batch things that are needed/wanted in one place the night before. This usually involves placing necessary items in a tote bag that hangs near the garage door. I also bunch things in the fridge together with a lunch box sitting on the counter as a visual reminder for myself to fill it.

When my son was doing therapies after school, I would bring a little cooler in my car that contained sparkling water, still water, juice boxes and an ice pack to keep things cold. I also had a lunch box that contained snack items for each of us. These two things didn't take more than 2 minutes to prepare and they helped reduce the urge to go through a fast food drive thru if I got hungry or thirsty. It also helped keep his blood sugar regulated since I never knew when he had last eaten.

Travels

I always map out the before, during and after of any trip that we are taking so that I know what is needed during each of those phases. I sit down with my notebook and use my Storyteller to mentally go through the travel process from locking the door and heading out to unlocking the door upon return. This helps me think about things like holding the mail, purchasing passes or tickets, booking reservations and grocery delivery scheduling. Because traveling is such an "out of routine" experience, having a written checklist to consult is a tension-reducing strategy that minimizes the pressure of having to rely on my memory to make sure all our bases are covered.

> Considering what works, what doesn't, and what we could do differently also plays a huge role in how we map out our days and activities.

This process has increased the ease and joy that I have around travel, which was something I used to dread. It also allows me to ask those I am traveling with about their wants and needs so that we can all be on the same page as much as possible.

**I wrote an ebook on this all - "Margaret Webb's Guide to Ease and Joy in Travel" - https://www.margaretwebblifecoach. com/ease-and-joy-in-travel.html.

Groceries

I enjoy mapping out our weekly meal plan. On Saturday or Sunday, I check in with family members to see what they might want/need from the store. I keep recipes in front of me so I can look in the freezer/fridge/pantry to see what I already have. When I'm ready to order, I know exactly what I need. I find it most convenient to utilize a grocery delivery service. Doing this might look more expensive because of the slight cost increase for items and the tipping that's required, but it really isn't since, for me (and I suspect most people), in-store shopping usually results in impulse buying of things I don't really need and duplicate buying of things I already have.

We have also started utilizing a grocery checklist for my son to fill out on Saturday when I place our grocery order. This process means that he has to go into the pantry, fridge and freezer to make sure he's got the food and drink he'd like to have for the week. We began doing this as a way to build the executive functioning skills necessary for greater independence and he is motivated to do it because if it's not on the list, I'm not buying it.

Holiday Seasons

Similar to traveling and grocery shopping, when it comes to the holidays, I map them out as well. Whether it is a one day celebration like Thanksgiving or the Super Bowl, or a whole season like Christmas, I think about my intention (and the intentions of those I will be with) in order to give attention to the things that are important to us - food, beverages, experiences, physical space arrangement, decorations, etc.

Again, I use the three questions to reflect on past experiences in order to use what we know that works for us, like having foods that my son will eat. It also helps us to figure out something different to try for those times when things didn't go as well, like reconsidering our expectations for including our son at the dinner table when foods have strong smells that are aversive to him.

All of these situations where I am mapping out what I can do to set myself (and my family) up for success only take between 5-20 minutes, unless I do a deep dive to tackle what comes up. Doing a deep dive during the mapping exercise might involve asking myself the "future self" question...

What can I do to help my future self out?

This often reveals simple things that I can do that, while seemingly minor, actually wind up relieving a ton of stress and allowing for more ease. When I started to recognize this and use the "future self" question to my advantage, I realized it made a big difference to everyone involved. I am more prepared and feel much calmer because I've done all I can to take care of the things that I have influence over. It also means I have more energy to go with the flow of any "unexpecteds" that are bound to pop up at the last minute!

Chapter Twenty-Six

Empowering Force #3 - Intentional Parenting Using Archetypes

You may remember being introduced to the Warrior archetype and how it drains your energy when it is in shadow. This archetype gets a lot of attention and praise from society, as in "Warrior Mom" or "Mama Bear," but since it is often the only archetype that is employed at the early phases of a hero's journey in parenting, the constant use of this intense and focused energy leads to exhaustion.

Don't get me wrong, I've totally been both of these many, many times! The Warrior Mom and Mama Bear archetypes definitely have their time and place. But beware the shadow payoff of being in full-on Warrior mode all the time. I've noticed that, because of its recognized value by others, people come to view their Warrior energy as a badge of honor. It's as though they view the assertiveness (some might say aggressiveness) that characterizes the Warrior as the best and most obvious way to protect and support their child. But allow me to shed some light on how the overuse of the Warrior mode may not always be the best approach and can have unintended consequences surrounding those who are involved with our children.

Just for a moment step into and fully embrace the Warrior archetype as Parent/Caregiver. Feel the intensity. Feel the need to fight for and protect your child. Now imagine what it might feel like for a teacher, school counselor or therapist to have you walk into the room with this energy. Chances are extremely high that they are going to feel defensive before anything is said or done. They are going to be guarded and feel like they are being attacked.

You may be really upset because of some disturbing episode involving your child or because of a decision that negatively impacts the services they receive. That is totally understandable and like I said above, sometimes the Warrior is needed to set boundaries and enforce things.

However, I would encourage you to get curious about whether or not your Warrior needs to be as active as they are in your life. If you think about it, it takes a lot of energy to fight and defend constantly and I know people who've only backed off with the intensity only after getting sick or injured.

Instead, what has worked really well for me is to check in with my intention from the perspective of my Monarch/Elder. When presented with a challenge, I envision myself zooming out to create some energetic distance and get perspective around what is going on to see what would be best. I bring in my child archetype in order to tap into curiosity and say...

- I'm curious about...
- What do I notice about this?

It is also powerfully helpful to get curious about each person as well as the environment that is involved in the challenging situation.

> I know I've said this before but there really is so much good information that often gets overlooked when immediately jumping into Warrior mode!

Zooming out in the context of a behavior issue or academic difficulty can help you and those who work with your child come together to share and discuss these questions...

- What works for your child?
- What does not or is not working for your child?
- What are some things that you all can try to see if there is a better way for your child?

Imagine, if you can, your four archetypes standing alongside you, each one offering you their strengths at the just the right level in order to approach things in an effective and efficient manner. That is an awesome collaboration.

> The following was shared earlier but I think it is helpful to revisit them in detail for this section.

The Four Archetypes and their Shadow Descriptions:

The Child

The Child archetype is all about play, curiosity, learning and pursuing passions. It is helpful as it reminds me to be curious and to consider what my intention is for whatever I am doing. This archetype is not bound by doing what is known but is open to lots of possibilities and inspiration.

Too much of the Child archetype involves being too unrealistic about what is actually possible in a situation, not wanting to have or take any responsibility, jumping from one thing to another without following through and/or handing everything over to the "experts" without concern.

Too little of the Child archetype involves not being curious at all; having no joy or passion in one's life and feeling like one is wearing horse blinders with limited perspective.

The Warrior

The Warrior archetype is helpful in order to get stuff done and to set and protect boundaries. This archetype is focused on details, supporting and defending.

Too much of the Warrior archetype is being too forceful and defensive; having intense focus when it is not needed, always being busy doing/defending/protecting regardless of exhaustion and/or controlling.

Too little of the Warrior archetype looks like having no boundaries and allowing others to walk all over you, saying yes when you want to say no and not having clarity about the big picture which results in being wishy-washy.

The Teacher/Community Builder

I've taken some creative liberties here and call this one the Teacher/Community Builder because it seems to resonate best for the parents I coach. This archetype is focused on bringing people together to share, inform, as well as to celebrate and care for one another.

Too much of the Teacher/Community Builder archetype involves spending too much time trying to educate everyone whether or not they want to listen. Too much of this archetype may also look like needing others to agree with or do similar things you've decided to try in order to validate your choices.

Too little of the Teacher/Community Builder archetype looks like isolating oneself and feeling like you have to do everything yourself. There is often little trust that others will understand and not judge and also a feeling like you are never doing anything right and that everyone else knows better.

Monarch/Elder

The Monarch/Elder archetype is helpful in order to see the big picture of what is best. This archetype is able to take a step back, removing themselves from the drama of the past, present or future concerns in order to make decisions about what can be done or tried. The Monarch/Elder utilizes the experience and knowledge that they have and also employ the other archetypes to help them with their greater purpose.

Too much of the Monarch/Elder archetype looks like controlling and micromanaging everything as well as not being open to what others have to say unless they are deemed to be "experts."

Too little of the Monarch/Elder archetype involves not making any decisions, being wishy-washy about what to do, not trusting themselves to use the experience and knowledge that they have, but rather handing over power to others, even non-experts.

There may be times where there is resistance to change or someone might get defensive if they feel like they are part of the issue or problem. This is when stepping into the role of calm, yet assertive leader (Monarch/Elder along with Warrior) is helpful. You can express your wants and needs from a place of clarity without blame by going back to the intention of what is best for your child. It is times like this that make it really important to be clear on what your intention is before even going into a meeting.

One thing to keep in mind is that while you are the Leader for your child's team and have your intentions for what you are wanting, every person who you meet with has their own intention. Realizing this, if you notice tension arising, this is a wonderful time to tap into curiosity and simply inquire about that person's intention. They might just be doing what they have always done before or operating from their own internal rules about how students/clients/patients "should" be. Noticing and having curiosity can change the energy of the situation immediately.

This might feel awkward and uncomfortable at first but it is quite a powerful tool to help people to be clear on what they are wanting and why they are wanting it. You may discover that the intentions that you or the others involved have are not realistic or don't take into consideration who the child is or the environment that they are in. This is awesome to know and from there, shifts in the intentions can be made to more accurately reflect reality. This is all good to know and feels so good to me!!

Simply asking yourself, "Which archetype or archetypes would help me most in this situation?" can help you to find new ways of being a parent, ways that hopefully make you feel more empowered and allow for more peace, ease and joy. It can also help in almost every other aspect of your life. Good to know!

Chapter Twenty-Seven

Empowering Force #4 - Self Care

The hero's journey in parenting typically begins with exhaustion and you've been given tools throughout this book to help you relax the intense focus you've had on your child and start taking care of yourself by observing your stories and emotions in order to feel more calm and clear as a parent. Despite what you now know, unexpecteds will always pop up and therefore self-care becomes a critically Empowering Force for parenting!

You may notice that even the thought of taking care of yourself might activate your Warrior because it thrives in "doing" mode. You may become aware of some limiting and judgmental thoughts —"I don't have time for that" or "If I do x for myself, I'm not doing enough for my child." or "What will the other parents think if I'm doing x while they are doing y?"

> This is why I've shared what I have up to this point, so you can notice and question those thoughts, reassuring your

> Warrior that self care is actually going to help you be more of the parent you desire to be.

There seems to be an unspoken social rule that we must do everything for our children at all times, especially if the child experiences any sort of challenge, setting aside our own wants and needs until our children are grown and happy. This may have been an internal rule that was modeled for and taught to us as we grew up or it could be something that is conveyed throughout the parenting community.

I've seen many parents take pride in the fact that they are willing to forego their own self-care in order to sacrifice everything for their child. I've also seen parents who cannot do something for themselves without a tremendous amount of guilt *(Think of Kristin Bell's character at the beginning of the movie "Bad Moms.")* I also know many parents whose children are now adults with their own kids who still set their wants and needs aside because they feel like they "have to" take care of those adult children or their grandchildren.

Good to know AND I respectfully say that this is total BS for many reasons, but mainly because I've personally seen my son become happier and more self confident as I have become happier and more self confident. Sure, you can do all you can to support your child learning and growing AND you can take care of yourself. I've said it before and I'll say it again...

We are role models for our children about what it means and looks like to be an adult.

If we cannot allow ourselves to be happy and model caring for ourselves, what message are they getting about what is possible for them as adults?

The fact is that we cannot control if our children are going to be happy or not. You can do all sorts of things to try and make things go smoothly for them AND they might still throw a tantrum, have a meltdown, not appreciate what you have given or done for them, or they might have obstacles like anxiety or depression that make things challenging for them.

For us, the reality of having a child who is on his own developmental timeline is that he may live with us forever, as we aren't sure what level of independence he will have as an adult. What the future holds is a huge unknown and it doesn't have to mean that we resign to denying ourselves fun, relaxation and growth experiences in order to live a life that solely revolves around him. It means that our self care is important and becomes an Empowering Force allowing us to best support him.

Create Supportive Routines

My husband and I came to terms with this early on, back when he was 15 months old, not yet babbling, and testing began. While the possibility that he would not be independent wasn't ever something we considered prior to this time, we made the conscious decision that if that was the case, we wanted our lives to be as satisfying and enjoyable as possible, with us doing what we needed to do in order to be a team working together.

For us, that looked like creating routines and rituals in order to consistently have fun and stay connected as a couple and as a family.

> We have always been like that as a couple, even before becoming parents, so consider what works for you and your family and do that.

Here are some of our routines:

Friday Night Pizza Night

We love food so we do pizza dinners on Friday nights. We have our favorite delivery place or we make our own. Since our son doesn't like tomatoes he gets garlic bread or crust with just mozzarella cheese on it.

Once we are done eating, our son watches a show in his room while we watch a movie, usually a comedy because laughter is always a wonderful form of self-care!

Saturday Date Night at Home Dinner

My husband is an amazing chef and going out for dinner is more hassle than it is worth as we still need someone to come over and hang out with our son while we are gone. Because of this we have opted for at-home date night dinners on Saturday nights. We both love to cook and it is super fun to expand the repertoire of what we can make by preparing foods from around the globe, like Argentina, China, France, Germany, Italy, Japan, Korea, Mexico, Morocco, and Spain as well as favorites from around the United States.

Sunday Family Dinners and Family Movie Night

Grandma and Great Grandma come over for a pre-dinner game of Euchre and a dinner that they select, usually spaghetti, steak and mashed potatoes or pulled pork sandwiches and fries.

Once they leave, the three of us take turns selecting a Disney or Pixar movie from Disney+. This has helped our son become more flexible in watching something that he may not have picked and is something we are intentional about since he is an only child. Unless he was with his cousins, he usually got to pick whatever he wanted.

Some ways my husband and I have created more care for ourselves as parents:

- We found restaurants that had food that we all liked. We would go early so it wasn't crowded. With each one we routinely visited, we got to know the staff who all fell in love with our son, which helped tremendously when he wasn't having a great day.
- When we lived far from family members, we found people who were interested in education, occupational/speech therapy or social work to watch our son if we needed an evening out. There are also sitter services that are starting to be geared towards

those with special needs or who are neurodivergent.

- We planned getaways to do things that we knew he would love, local "staycations" to places like Hyatt Lost Pines as well as bigger trips to Disney World.
- We began taking ski trips to places like Park City and Telluride that had adaptive sports programs - NAC - National Ability Center in Park City and TASP - Telluride Adaptive Sports Program in Telluride. I had no idea that adaptive sports programs even existed before we were invited on a ski trip with good friends and it was wonderful!! We have had positive experiences each time and the people who work and volunteer for these places are there because they truly love what they do.
- We would invite grandparents to stay with him so that we could go on vacation without him. This was important for us to have something to look forward to and also create memories of our own.

Our routines and rituals have strengthened our connection with our son and it has helped us build our relationships with one another. We know this is a long journey that didn't end when he turned 18 last year. As I said earlier, he may always live with us and if so, we will continue to take care of ourselves so that we can care for one another.

I also realize that quite often on parenting journeys like ours, relationships and partnerships can be challenged to the point where they aren't salvageable or healthy for those involved. For some, parenting alone can make things easier. For others, it can make things harder. If you are parenting alone or co-parenting, self care is still important and just might look different from homes where tag-teaming is a possibility.

There were many days when I was exhausted and my husband was working and so we implemented "Rest Time" and my son would sit on the bed with me to watch a DVD while I closed my eyes. There were also times when I would lay on the floor in his room while he looked at ceiling fan catalogs and I closed my eyes.

Putting Your Own Mask On First

Creating family connections is important but so is something that is stated on every airplane ride: "Put on your own oxygen mask first before assisting others." Why? Because you are NO help to anyone else if you don't have your own oxygen or energy.

I'm going to assume that you have experienced some level of placing everyone's needs above your own. You might even have a good understanding about what happens as a result and if you aren't sure how it affects you, begin by noticing how you feel when you are doing everything for everyone else. Is there an undercurrent of energy filled with resentment, frustration, spite, irritation, annoyance, etc.? *(Remember how I felt that Sunday as I cleaned the kitchen while everyone else was enjoying a relaxing morning? That is what I'm talking about!!)* Is this how you want to feel? Is this how you want to care for those you love?

Most people would probably say that they want their family life to be happy, loving, relaxed, enjoying time together and creating memories. Isn't it ironic that we end up creating the opposite of what we desire to have because of an idea that it is selfish to take care of ourselves?

Self care can take a million different forms, but it is simply taking care of your physical and emotional needs. When I am exhausted, overwhelmed and doing too much without refueling my own energy, I am no good to anyone and am definitely not the mother or wife that I want to be. When I notice this (usually sparked by a feeling of irritation or annoyance or thought that someone else "should" be doing something different), I press pause, get still and ask myself...

What do I want or need right now?

This simple question offers up so much wisdom to help me in that moment. It shifts everything because instead of things happening TO me, I am now empowering myself to do something different.

When the concept of self care is tossed out, most people jump to the assumption that it means a day at the spa or a week-long vacation. Not so! Don't get me wrong, I always appreciate those opportunities, but asking myself what I am wanting or needing when I notice those feelings creep in is always fascinating.

Take a minute and ask yourself what YOU are wanting or needing at this moment.

If you are new to this, you may notice that the first things that pop into your mind are things that you could do for your family. Just take a breath and ask yourself again, "What am I wanting or needing right now?"

- *It might be something that brings you joy like sipping on a delicious coffee or listening through earbuds to YOUR music (not Kids Bop or Radio Disney) while driving your children to their activities.*
- *It might be a phone call to a friend who makes you laugh.*
- *It might be a hug, a nap or five minutes to yourself. (There have been many times I've gone to the bathroom simply to have some time alone and even if there were little fingers appearing under the door. I did what I could to take some deep breaths in order to regroup before opening the door.)*
- *It might be noticing an emotion that you didn't even realize was there wanting to be felt and released. (As I mentioned earlier, the Guardian of the Heart likes to protect you from feeling emotions AND releasing stored emotions can be a wonderful form of self care.)*

If this is something you haven't allowed for yourself in a while, I strongly encourage you to create a list or menu of things that help you to refuel and recharge. It was helpful for me because I was so used to NOT giving myself what I needed or wanted that having something I could refer to when my mind went blank despite knowing I desperately needed something helped tremendously.

At first, it felt really uncomfortable, as though it was selfish and like I was trying to get away with something or like I was breaking some sort of parenting law. Funny, right?! Or maybe you can relate. Regardless, I can honestly say that my family has truly benefited from me taking care of myself.

I no longer carry around that undercurrent of energy filled with exhaustion, annoyance, frustration or irritation and if I do notice it emerging, I know what to do! I also feel really good about encouraging them to care for themselves by doing what they want and need so it goes both ways.

Margaret's Self Care Menu:

- taking some deep breaths
- a long, hot shower
- 5 minutes of quiet
- Sunday afternoon nap
- husband taking over when our son is stuck on something and I'm losing my patience with him
- date night

- night alone at nearby hotel
- a good cry
- coffee in my favorite buffalo plaid mug
- getting a massage
- pjs at 5 pm
- takeout or DoorDash for dinner
- grocery shopping alone or utilizing grocery delivery service like Instacart
- a hug
- listening to a podcast that resets my thinking
- watching a favorite show or movie
- doing nothing
- spending a weekend morning purging and decluttering
- a glass of wine while chatting with a faraway friend
- listening to music that feels like me even if it is through my earbuds
- dancing and singing into a wooden spoon while making dinner

What sorts of self care things would be on your menu?

Chapter Twenty-Eight

Empowering Force #5 - Gratitude

Our children are the reason behind our hero's journey in parenting and are wonderful teachers for us all. As you may have noticed at the beginning of this book, gratitude was not the defining feature of my early parenting experiences! I think it is rare for anyone who has an "unexpected" plopped into their life to be able to shift into a perspective of gratitude immediately, welcoming with open arms all of the challenges facing us and the demanding lessons those challenges bring.

Leap-frogging over underlying Shadow and Hindering Forces can be done, but from what I've experienced, it doesn't get you very far on your journey. I initially fought and resisted the necessary shifts in expectations that I had for what I thought parenting was going to be like. This only resulted in an undercurrent of energy that felt dissonant. While I wanted more ease and joy in parenting, I felt frustration and resentment because things weren't easy and I couldn't always access joy when I compared our life and our experiences with others.

Using the tools I have shared to process my thoughts and emotions in a healthy manner, I was able to get to a place where I truly feel grateful. It is because of my child and a willingness to acknowledge that there were (and still are) so many things he was able to teach me, that I am the *me* I am today.

I am grateful for all that I have learned and because of this unexpected twist in life, I now know things about myself that I didn't know before...or had simply forgotten. I am a more open, curious, compassionate and patient person and parent. I have learned to give myself permission to love what I love without apology just like my son does with his own passions.

I'm grateful for all of the connections I now have with others on this journey. I have been teaching and coaching for over twelve years and I am not only able to share what has been helpful for me and what I've actually done, I get to be on this hero's journey in parenting with many other amazing parents.

Gratitude to Empower You During Challenging Times

Gratitude is a tool that not only shines a light on more obvious things to be thankful for, it also helps the Storyteller to re-pattern the thinking mind from searching for the negative, which it does quite easily as it scans for danger, to looking for the positive in any given situation.

Sometimes finding gratitude when situations are particularly challenging is tough so here are two of my favorite Gratitude Empowering Force questions that I turn to...

- *What is perfect about this?*
- *What is this trying to teach me or help me practice?*

"What's perfect about this?" isn't about how something is ideal but rather about finding something, anything, that can shift the perspective from being a victim of circumstance to one of a curious and empowered problem solver. There is always something that is perfect in any given situation and viewing it from the lens of these questions feels so much better.

While there are way too many situations to share here where this question has helped me to reframe, there is one particular situation that stands out in my mind.

Example:

One morning, I came out of my bedroom and smelled a very potent smell of different spices. I walked into the kitchen and saw the culprit...several spice jars had been emptied into a cast iron pan that was sitting on the stove. The lids of the jars were on the counter along with all but one of the jars.

My son loves to spin and can spin pretty much anything. He was always trying to spin my glass spice jars but I told him he couldn't because they were full of spices. He fixed that by removing the spices.

As I looked at the mishmosh of dried spices in the pan, including some fairly pricey ones like turmeric and curry, I asked myself, "What's perfect about this?"

- *It was perfect because he had dumped them into a contained space and not all over the floor so I didn't have to contend with the dog ingesting something that could be toxic for him.*

- *It was perfect because for someone like him with a heightened sense of smell, I think he got a natural consequence from the intense smell of cumin, coriander, cayenne, curry and turmeric.*

- *It was perfect because nothing broke and he didn't get hurt.*

- *It was perfect because while expensive, spices can be easily replaced.*

- *It was also perfect and a bit humorous because he took what I said literally and didn't spin the jar with spice in it but took care of that obstacle for himself.*

He was probably quite proud that he solved that problem and got what he wanted!

Can you see how simply asking, "What's perfect about this?" creates a shift? It works by helping to shift the thinking mind away from the ever-present negative evidence toward the connecting compassion of a more positive perspective. Had I focused on how this sucked, I would have been annoyed for much longer.

I absolutely had my, "Are you freaking kidding me?!?" and "Ughhhh!" moment but cycled through those thoughts and feelings pretty fast. It all got cleaned up within 5 minutes, replacements were purchased, he was given one jar to spin while being explicitly told that the ones in the drawer were mine and were not spinners, empty or full. It was perfect in that it reminded me that he needs to have that specificity.

People email and text me all of the time asking, "Alright Margaret, what's perfect about *this* situation?" and it often involves them having a perfect opportunity to practice...

- Setting boundaries
- Saying "No"
- Reconnecting with intention and doing what actually matters in the moment
- Asking for support
- Allowing for some self care
- Remembering that you cannot control another human being

- Remembering that jumping into someone else's business or strong emotional energy is not helpful because you can notice so much more that is effective when not in their business or joining them in their energy

Asking "What's perfect about this?" is one way into gratitude when it is not immediately apparent. I encourage you to play with this and see if it helps bring more lightness into those annoying things that are bound to pop up in parenting while also helping you to cycle through them faster. This also helps to model for our children that unexpected things happen, they aren't the end of the world and it's much better to see how we can learn from them than getting stuck in anger and frustration when something undesirable inevitably happens.

Everyday Gratitude

Taking time for gratitude isn't something that should just be done on special occasions or holidays. Noticing and expressing gratitude on a regular basis is another way to repattern the Storyteller's perspective from searching for the negative to an awareness of all sorts of things, big and small, to be grateful for.

Here are some of my favorite gratitude primers...

- I love it when...
- I am grateful for this piece of clothing item because

it makes me feel...

- I love the season of x because...
- I am grateful for this food or beverage because...
- I am grateful for this kind of music or musician because...
- My favorite flower is x because...
- I love this scent because it reminds me of...
- My favorite time of day is x because...
- I love looking at this color because when I do I feel...
- I love using this writing instrument because...
- I am grateful for these things that make life easier...
- I enjoy this particular creative outlet because...
- Doing this physical activity makes me so happy because it makes me feel...
- This is my favorite movie because it reminds me...
- I love this particular space in my home because...
- I am grateful for this person because...

When I began doing this it was like a window shade opened for me and I began noticing more and more things that made my heart happy. I would just comment out loud while driving to school or therapy sessions about the beautiful sunrises, sunsets or cloud formations.

For a while I didn't know if my son was paying attention but it didn't matter. I was soaking them in and then one day, we were driving somewhere and he made the funniest sounding utterance and made a comment about the sky. He was making in his own way the sound I made when I would say, "Ahhhhhh...look at the beautiful sky!" Made me laugh and also made me realize that what I was doing was making a difference.

Play with practicing gratitude and see the difference that allowing yourself to notice little bits of love, joy and gratitude can do to lift your spirits, even on days that are filled with challenges.

Expressing Gratitude

I thought I'd share something that I've been noticing with my son lately...he appreciates being appreciated. Don't we all?

As someone who does a ton for the other people in my life, it feels good to have someone say, "Thank you for doing that!" Because I notice the difference in how it feels to be appreciated, I've been trying to make a point to express my genuine gratitude for my son doing things even if it is something that he was asked to do. (Genuine gratitude is important as sarcastic insincere gratitude defeats the purpose. Our children know and feel the difference.)

I express gratitude when he brings up his laundry basket and places it just inside of the laundry room. "Thanks for bringing your laundry basket up! That is a huge help."

I express gratitude when he puts his plate in the sink. "Oh my gosh! Thank you so much for putting your dish in the sink and not leaving it on the counter. That is so helpful!!"

I express gratitude when he closes the garage door after his bike ride. "Hey, you closed the garage door after your bike ride! That is so awesome and helps to make sure that your bike doesn't get stolen because that would be so unexpected and disappointing!"

Why do I do this? I do it because I think oftentimes the focus can be on what is not done and over time, that becomes frustrating. Imagine the same scenario with these as my responses (or lack thereof)...

"Why didn't you just put your laundry basket all the way in the laundry room. It was literally four more steps."

"The dishwasher had space. I'm not sure why you didn't just put your dishes in there instead of putting them in the sink."

I could say nothing about closing the garage door and not draw attention to something he did that was really important.

Add on developmental, physical or executive functioning challenges and one can easily adopt a "why bother" attitude since nothing is ever done "good enough."

> This isn't just our children! It is our partners and caregiving team as well who can take on this attitude of "If I can't do it like he/she/they want, why bother?!"

I don't want that. I want to encourage him to do what he can and to let him know that I notice what he is doing because it probably took him a lot of mental energy to remember to do the thing in the first place.

This doesn't mean that I don't support him in growing towards the next step of the task he has done but my energy around it is totally different. It is not an energy of annoyance, it is one of gratitude that he did something at all and from there I can say something like,

"Thank you so much for bringing your laundry to the laundry room! It is so helpful to have it there and maybe next time if the washer is empty, you can put your clothes in there and start it. Do you remember how to do this or do you want me to show you? You can also let me know and I will help you. I bet it felt really good to get all of those dirty clothes and towels out of your bedroom."

He usually says something like, "Thanks!" and maybe, "There are always things in the washer and it's really annoying to have mom's stuff in there when I try to do my laundry." (Keeping things real here!)

I could be equally as annoyed that he said something like this but it probably is annoying for him since I usually do leave our clothes or towels in there. I agree with him and reiterate that I'm just so happy that he brought them up and will do what I can to help him in the future.

Shifting the focus from what our children aren't doing or what they aren't able to do yet to expressing gratitude for what they do feels better for all involved as far as I'm concerned. It also can create an energy of willingness to do things because, like I said earlier, it just feels good to be appreciated for what one does...no matter how big or small it may be. Try it (or continue doing it) and notice the difference it makes in your everyday life.

Chapter Twenty-Nine

Empowering Force #6 - Actively Seeking and Creating Joy

When times get hard and things aren't going the way we expected, joy is typically the first thing that is eliminated. This usually happens because there are all sorts of thoughts and stories (thanks Storyteller!) that we tell ourselves about what it means about us as parents if we are happy while our child is unhappy or showing worrisome signs of developmental delays and is not doing what their chronological peers are doing.

There can also be a strong response from our Warrior who is trying to protect us from feeling disarmed when something doesn't go as expected and so it can feel safer to live in tension, but is that how you want to live life? Having lived that way for years I can honestly say that it doesn't have to be like that.

When your life begins to feel as though joy is no longer attainable, it becomes necessary to begin questioning thoughts like, "It is selfish to want time for myself when my child still needs support." or "The minute I allow myself to relax and/or have fun, the phone is going to ring or I will get a text about my child."

Questioning these joy-robbing thoughts begins by asking yourself if they represent the actual truth of the situation or are they simply reflecting your fears and insecurities. Convince yourself that you can disown these negative thoughts by imagining more positive turnaround examples that show how the opposite can be equally true with better outcomes for all involved.

Try to remember those times when something you feared would happen, didn't occur. It's not easy to remember those times since our memory is not really geared toward storing non-events, but I'm convinced that fearing negative outcomes that never materialize happens more often than we realize.

These negative thoughts and fearful imaginings are hindrances to joy. But they can be overcome by reminding ourselves that we are not our thoughts and trying to control the outcome of events before they occur is impossible and, ultimately, counterproductive.

I am also realistic and know how challenging this can be at times so these questions help bring me into the present moment, even if only for a moment...

Can I allow for joy anyways knowing I can only do something about what happens only when/if it happens?

If I have a sense that something is probably going to happen, can I soak up the time that I've got to feel a little joy?

Self-care in its various forms is essential for parents and caregivers and hopefully what I've shared so far has gotten you on the path to having more energy and feeling less exhausted and overwhelmed. Now let's go a bit deeper and learn ways to intentionally and actively create a form of self care that is always an intention of mine - to have more joy in life!

When thinking about actively seeking joy, you may imagine a month-long vacation on a remote island drinking fruity concoctions from pineapples while being massaged. Sure, that would be lovely, but personally, I had to learn how to weave joy into my everyday life in the smallest of ways. Honestly, having grand thoughts about what I "should" do to have more joy in my life resulted in overwhelming anxiety which was NOT what I wanted or needed. Finding joy in the simple things not only got the snowball of change going, it quickly made a huge difference.

For me, simple things that bring me joy are...

- seeing and using my favorite plaid reusable "Unpaper Towels"
- sitting under a favorite blanket
- listening to a podcast that makes me laugh out loud
- smelling the sleepy corn chip puppy smell that comes from my dogs when they snuggle with me.

Now it is time for you to get curious about what brings YOU joy - not members of your family! Allowing yourself to ponder this can help you to intentionally cultivate joy and allow it into your life. Knowing what brings you joy can help you make any aspect of your life better. This is especially true for those times or experiences that aren't your favorite, like errands, school drop-off/pickup, therapy waiting rooms, etc.

I find that the perfect place to start is through something we almost always have access to...our senses. Checking in with your senses might feel really basic but it really is a wonderful way to explore what makes you happy without filtering it through your thinking mind.

Chapter Thirty

Sensing Your Way to Joy Through Sight

This is the sense we are most connected to yet probably use it mostly to judge or gather information. Let's try something different and use this sense to gather some more joyful information.

Have you ever taken some time to really connect with what you love to look at? What colors, shapes, patterns, flowers, things, etc. draw you to them? What sort of architecture or design do you love? Are you drawn to settings with minimal visual stimulation? Do you love the rich visual appeal of some favorite setting in your home? Everyone is different and this is simply a way to start connecting with what YOU love.

I was so disconnected from what brought me joy that I had to start from square one, wandering through the grocery store, a bookstore or an arts and crafts store and just noticing what caught my attention in a good way. I didn't have to buy anything. I would just take a deep breath and soak in the good feelings that come from something small, like the color of a fruit or vegetable or a plaid pattern on a tissue box. Again, I didn't have to purchase these things in order to get joy from them. Snapping a photo or just noticing them brought me moments of joy.

If this sounds fun and you still aren't sure what brings you joy OR if you want more ideas, wander through stores with the intention to notice what catches your attention. You can also play with gathering up catalogs or magazines and tearing out the pages that have words or images that bring you joy. Frame them individually or create a collage and place them around your home in places where you spend the most time. This is a wonderful way to connect with your joy throughout the day and it only takes a second.

I remember that when I first began doing this, I was shocked by how much joy I received from looking at postcards of a pumpkin, sunflower, and autumn leaves. I framed them and they continue to bring me joy every time I look at them.

Simple things that bring me joy to look at:

- Almost any plaid pattern
- Autumn colors
- Roses and sunflowers
- Sunrises and sunsets
- Papermate Flair pens in a mason jar

Think about what brings YOU joy to look at and find small ways of incorporating them into your everyday life so you can get little plug-ins of joy throughout your day!

> I am intentionally NOT tying joy with family even though they can absolutely provide it. I want you to focus on YOU and what brings you joy independent of other people.

Chapter Thirty-One

Sensing Your Way to Joy Through Smell

Smell is such an interesting and powerful sense as it seems to capture memories. I am taken back in time whenever I smell the scents of an automotive repair garage as it reminds me of my dad who started his career as a mechanic before building an automotive parts/service business. I have such specific memories of visiting him when I was a young child and also of the time I spent working for him as a young adult.

Considering the power this sense has, when was the last time you took time to truly smell things that you use all of the time, like soap, shampoo, candles, dish soap, perfume, deodorant, etc? Do you ever take a second to soak in the delicious smells of the food that you are cooking or the wine, tea or coffee that you are drinking?

We can also get so used to smells in our everyday lives that even if we love them, unless we consciously focus on them, they can go unnoticed.

I used to be very disconnected from my sense of smell, which is surprising because it is actually a really powerful sense for me. When I got curious about this, I discovered that I wasn't smelling because I wasn't in the present moment. I was busy in my mind re-living or pre-living experiences, so unless it was an unusual or incredibly strong odor that came my way, I didn't pay attention to it.

As I began my joy-seeking explorations I discovered that despite using a certain brand of shampoo and soap for years, I actually hated the way they smelled. I wasn't one to spend a lot of money on things like this so I typically bought products that my husband and I could both use. I had long hair and had to laugh about the fact that I was surrounded by something that actually made me quite agitated. After that realization, I spent a good deal of time in the shampoo and soap aisle, carefully choosing products that made me happy. I now choose scents based on the seasons and love finding new "flavors" (as my son calls the scents) that make me happy.

While I have always loved the scents of certain perfumes, wearing them was one of the things that I had let go of because of my son's sensory sensitivities as well as those who were at his therapy offices. I think we've all been in a situation where we found it intensely jarring to be in the presence of someone who went a little too heavy with their perfume or cologne.

As I began reconnecting with what joy felt like for me, I revisited my favorite perfumes and allowed myself to smell them. I realized I didn't have to give them up 100% and started to enjoy them without spraying them on myself. Sometimes I would spray them onto a cotton ball and place them in an old spice jar or baggie. I'd put this in my purse to smell if I wanted to connect with a certain feeling state that the scent evoked. I also spray them in my bathroom sink so that I can enjoy the scent without it overpowering the whole house. This is how I create just a little joy for myself when I am washing my hands or getting myself ready in the morning.

**If you do the sink thing, brush your teeth first unless you want perfume in your mouth.

Essential oils are also a really fun way to play with scents. I now have a baggie filled with my favorite small bottles and when I know I am going into a situation that might bring up anxiety, I pull out my Balsam Fir and Lavender bottles and just breathe them in. This immediately calms my body and mind.

My Favorite Smells:

- Butter, garlic and shallots slowly simmering in a pan
- Star Jasmine
- Fresh cut grass
- Balsam Fir candle
- Mrs. Meyer's Lemon Verbena cleaning supplies
- Sleepy puppy smell
- Freshly laundered sheets and towels
- The entry ways of the Grand Floridian and Polynesian hotels in Disney World

Get curious and allow yourself to spend the few seconds it takes to tune into your sense of smell.

- What do YOU love to smell?
- What scent calms you?
- Empowers you?
- Reminds you of a favorite vacation?
- Feels comforting?

How can you allow for these in your everyday life?

Chapter Thirty-Two

Sensing Your Way to Joy Through Taste

When was the last time that you took a bite of something delicious and just savored the flavors? When was the last time you made a meal that you love the taste of because it is your favorite? Do you even remember what your favorite tastes are? Do you allow yourself to have and savor them?

I ask these questions because looking back to early on in my own journey, all too often I was shoveling food into my mouth without even paying attention to what it tasted like. I'd snack on food that I didn't even like simply because it was on my son's plate. I would prepare meals for us and be so focused on him and what he was doing that before I knew it, my plate was empty. I didn't even notice what it tasted like.

No more, because the reality is that I seriously love food!! Now, I take my time with the sensory experience of eating. I love taking a bite of something delicious, closing my eyes and just allowing myself to savor the flavors. I try to make sure that I am sitting down while I eat and try to taste each bite rather than devouring it in 2.9 seconds.

Some of my favorite foods are...

- Homemade "Juicy Lucy" Cheeseburger on a Brioche bun with pickles
- Eggs Benedict
- Holy Basil Chicken or Panang Curry and Rice
- Roast Beef Sandwich with Provolone and Kosher Pickles
- Spicy Tuna Sushi Roll with Wasabi and Ginger Soy Sauce
- Chicken and Mushroom Risotto
- Chicken Parmesan with Fresh Mozzarella
- Mexican Rice Bowl with Fresh Salsa and Guacamole
- Truffle Gouda
- Pumpkin Pie with Whipped Cream
- Cheesecake
- Chocolate Chip Cookie Dough Ice Cream

Take some time to think about what you love to taste and find ways to allow yourself to savor the flavors of them.

Chapter Thirty-Three

Sensing Your Way to Joy Through Touch

One of the things that the Battle Ready Bodyguard does is to try and protect oneself from feeling attacked and oftentimes that results in a disconnection from feeling comfortable in one's own body. I've shared some strategies earlier to support getting back to a place where, if disconnected, you can start small to feel things against your skin like noticing how clothes feel on your body or how wind feels on your cheeks.

> If you have experienced trauma, I encourage working with a trained professional. I am not a therapist or psychiatrist and these are simply suggestions I have employed to support finding joy through the use of my senses.

Every morning I typically determine what I want to wear starting with my socks. I love socks that are comfortable. I also love socks that support the mood I am in and the energy that I have that day. The type, color and/or pattern I choose helps me pick out the outfit that I wear. I don't know if I have super sensitive feet but it makes me really happy when I put on the pair I've chosen.

As I began reconnecting with myself and what brought me joy, I noticed my sense of touch more and more. While sitting outside on a summer evening, I would soak in the feeling of a cool-ish breeze coming through the trees. When it gets cold enough, nothing makes me happier than being chilly and feeling the warmth coming from a fire in the fireplace or fire pit.

My friend June gave me a cashmere blanket and there is nothing better than having that softness over my lap, keeping me cozy as I do coaching sessions or having it next to my face while I sleep. (Unfortunately my female dog shares my love of this blanket so I have less room on my side of the bed.) It makes me feel loved and content that I bring it with me when I travel. It goes in my carry-on so I've got it on the plane and now one of my favorite gifts to other people is a cashmere blanket.

Think about what you are putting on your body and feeling against your skin - socks, clothes, blankets, temperature, etc. Do they feel good and make you happy? Do they conjure up positive feeling states for you? It can be really helpful to create a list of the things that you love to touch so that you can be more intentional and aware to include more of them in your everyday life.

Here are some of my favorites...

- cashmere blanket
- soft socks
- down comforter
- grass under my feet
- open sunroof on a brisk morning
- super soft pjs
- flannel
- worn jeans
- warmth of a fire on a cold evening

Now go explore for yourself!! Add more of what feels good and subtract what doesn't.

Chapter Thirty-Four

Sensing Your Way to Joy Through Sound

This is an interesting sense because it is so unique to each individual. Some people like lots of noise or background sounds to help them feel good. Others enjoy silence. Sometimes certain music resonates and other times it doesn't. The differences in the way people respond to the wide variety of sounds that surround us is fascinating to me and I find myself super curious about the way sounds, in all their varied forms, bring people joy.

Do you find yourself listening to your kids music or videos while driving, even when they aren't in the car with you? I certainly did! I had nursery rhymes and Disney CDs playing in my car non-stop (This was pre-satellite radio, Spotify and Pandora and I'm sure Kidz Bop or Disney radio would be on if it existed back then!). Looking back on it, I don't even know if my son enjoyed listening to them and perhaps that's why he now loves driving in silence with me!

If someone had asked me what I love listening to, I would've drawn a complete blank. Me? What do I love listening to? I have no idea! Fortunately one of my coach friends asked me this question and I began an auditory exploration to figure this out.

Thank goodness for the apps that we have access to these days. I came to create stations, playlists and libraries filled with different kinds of music and podcasts to fit whatever mood I am in.

Some personal favorite Pandora and Spotify stations are Jack Johnson (great music for singing along while doing chores), Kelly Clarkson or Katy Perry (when I need some girl power energy), Bebel Gilberto (Great Brazilian music to make dinner to), Stan Getz (evening music), Acoustic New Age or Cozy Mornings (start the day music), Meditation or White Noise Radio (when I need to concentrate or focus on something).

I've found some great apps along my journey to help me when I need a little something extra due to stress, anxiety or other challenges. A favorite of mine is the BrainWave app. I use this when I need some super focused energy or if I am feeling anxious about something. It plays ambient noise and binaural waves and always seems to help me.

The Insight Timer app, introduced to me by my friend Kelley Wolf, is my go to when I am feeling distracted. The singing bowl sound immediately brings me back to the present moment. I can select the sound I want and have it go off in different time increments depending on how often I want or need to be brought back to the here and now.

The Calm app is something I love, too. It has sleep stories that I can listen to as I fall asleep. This isn't for everyone, especially if you are the kind of person who needs to hear the ending, like my son or husband. I am not one of those people and have yet to find out what happens on any of the train journeys I've listened to!

I also have podcasts that I love to listen to while cleaning the kitchen, prepping dinner or doing other daily chores. Favorites are Armchair Expert, Smartless, Fly on the Wall, Nobody's Listening, Right? and Differently Wired which is hosted by my good friend and colleague Debbie Reber.

I am not a big *sit down and read* a book kind of reader during the day. In fact, I haven't read any parenting books in years in part due to PTSD from the early ones I read way back when. But I also intentionally avoided parenting books when I began writing this book ten years ago because I didn't want them to influence what I wrote. I do love to listen to any Alexander McCall Smith book from any of his series while I walk the dogs.

Silence is another thing that I love. There are many times when my husband comes home and he wonders why there isn't any music playing. He loves music and while I do too, there are times when I prefer the silence. This is usually after a day of listening to my son say the same thing over and over again or answering endless questions about things I really don't remember or know about —like ceiling fans, outdoor light sconces or specific dates. Silence can be so wonderful!!

> Having wireless earbuds or headphones has been a game changer especially since I used to get the cord caught on a variety of things and the earbuds would get yanked out of my ears which never felt great.

Now onto YOU! What do YOU love to listen to? Create some stations, playlists and libraries just for you. Put some earbuds in your purse so you can listen whenever. Check out Audible to see if there are any books you'd love to listen to while grocery shopping or folding laundry or driving to/from work. Download some episodes of your favorite podcasts so that you can connect with the part of you that loves to learn, laugh, be inspired, etc. Have fun!!

Chapter Thirty-Five

Martha Beck's Three B's: Better It, Barter It, or Bag It

While there are many other minor rituals and routines that we've created with my son, the following are the more significant ones for me as a parent. When I began this journey in parenting, I did not feel these were possible and I now realize that my own self care is just as important as the care I give my son.

Give yourself a gift of joy and play with connecting with your senses and what YOU love, what brings YOU joy, even if it's even in tiny doses. It can make a huge difference!

People often resist allowing things that better their lives because they have thoughts and stories that this is selfish. These thoughts usually revolve around not having the time/money/energy for joy. But truly something as simple as a coffee, a chat with a friend, a glitter pen, a certain photograph or soft socks can bring tremendous amounts of joy!

I will be super annoying and say this again because it is really important...

We are role models for our children of what it means to be an adult!

Model for them that you can be a parent AND be happy, independent of them. The more you do this, the more natural it will feel even if it doesn't feel that way right now. Doing this will spread joy to all those you encounter and let them know that they too have permission to allow joy in their lives.

If you've been out of touch with who YOU are and what YOU want and need, create a collage of pictures and phrases that make you happy to look at. It's not necessarily about "things" you'd like to have, but more about creating the feeling state you get when looking at an image or phrase.

You can learn a lot about me from the collages I've made over the years. I love the colors of autumn and the contrast of cold snow and cozy interiors. This was another thing I picked up from reading Martha Beck's The Joy Diet. It is always amazing to me how simply looking at my collage can change my mood and energy. It also has led to small change after small change in my life that has made me happier. This makes me WAY more fun to be around as a mother and wife!

I can hear it now and have heard it from a lot of other moms - *"This is all great but I have kids and they have busy schedules so..."*

I totally understand and had similar thoughts until I learned about a tool from Martha Beck. I'm not sure what she calls it now but back then it was the "The 3 B's" - Bag It. Barter It. Better It." tool. It really helped me to empower myself to be more intentional around what I was doing in my everyday life and the decisions that I was making.

B #1 - "Bag It" involves choosing not to do things that are not important at the moment, or ever. Try looking at the list of things that you have on your "to-do" list. Consciously choose to not do the things that are draining and unnecessary. This means you'll have to get comfortable with saying no.

Learning to say "no" was incredibly challenging for me, so I had to find ways to do it in a way that felt good. I made it a habit to not agree to any commitments until I gave myself time to think about it. I also would look at my calendar to see if it was doable and realistic. This helped me play with getting comfortable saying, "No." or saying, "This isn't a good fit for us right now."

B #2 - "Barter It" is realizing that there are many possible ways to get necessary things done. Bartering involves acknowledging that there are things that I am good at and there are things that are not in my wheelhouse. I have found ways to allow other people to support me to get things off of my plate. This could be paying someone to clean the house, do laundry (I didn't realize this was an option and had a neighbor who did this and loved it!), walk dogs, organize things to create ease, etc.

Bartering doesn't have to involve money! You may find someone who loves to walk your dog. In exchange, you barter with them by helping them declutter spaces in their home, something you love to do and also something they've been wanting to do but cannot get motivated to do so.

When my son was younger, we had a babysitter who would either drive him to or pick him up from school so that I didn't have to do both 30 minute one way drives. She needed money as she was about to start grad school and was also about to be a new mom. I was starting my business and I needed time. It was a win-win situation for both of us.

There are people who love doing the most random things. There are people who offer lice management services after all! So, if there is something on your plate that you don't want to do but know that it needs to be done, get curious to see if there is a barter option possible and put it out there! If money is tight, you never know if you have a special skill that another person needs who also has a skill that you need.

B #3 - "Bettering It" is when you do what you can to better the situation. If there is a task that you need to do but aren't super crazy about doing it, incorporating ways to better it, even in the smallest of ways, can make a huge difference in the overall experience.

I used to hate going to my son's speech therapy sessions until I began stopping at the coffee shop and getting an iced latte to sip on while I sat at a picnic table outside of the office. I would catch up on emails and if the weather wasn't great, I'd sit in my car chatting with my sister. This shifted a previously dreaded experience into one that I started looking forward to.

As parents and caregivers, there are always going to be things that we choose to do for our children that may not be the most fun for us (carpool, sports practices, waiting rooms, etc.). This doesn't mean that these things have to be completely unpleasant. If you choose to do something, do what you can to make it as pleasant as possible.

I learned that by adding some things that I really enjoyed or wanted to do, I began to look at things previously dreaded, like time in the waiting room, driving carpool, etc. as a gift. These were now moments of time where I got to do something for myself instead of feeling trapped in an annoying situation. Allowing yourself to add things that make you happy creates such a different attitude and you get to be more YOU!

> This still applies when you have multiple children. It just requires a little more thought and planning but it is still possible to better any situation even if it means starting small.

Things I've added to add joy and better my everyday life:

- Audio books and podcasts
- An Ember coffee cup that keeps my coffee warm until I finish it
- Flowers from the grocery store placed in mason jars throughout my home
- Headphones – noise canceling earbuds or airpods

- Brain Wave, Calm, and Insight Timer apps
- iPhone/iPad with my favorite music, movies or apps.
- Favorite pen/pencil and journal to write thoughts, ideas, lists, etc.
- Coloring book for adults
- A beverage – flavored sparkling water is my favorite these days
- Favorite catalogs or magazines
- Needlepoint or cross stitch project (so meditative for me!!)

What are some things that bring YOU joy?

What are some ways you can utilize the 3 B's (Bag it. Barter it. Better it.) to support yourself?

Part Six Conclusion: Summary, Key Concepts and Power Questions

Summary:

I hope that the Empowering Forces I have shared with you have inspired you not only to give yourself permission to allow for curiosity, gratitude and joy in your life, but to also prioritize them in order to model for your child/children that they are important and can be different for everyone. They can also help you shift how you are feeling even when it has been a challenging day.

Key Concepts:

- Creating Balanced Flow Using Natural Energy Cycle
- Setting Myself Up for Success
- Intentional Parenting Using Archetypes
- Self Care
- Gratitude
- Actively Seeking and Creating Joy

Power Questions:

- How can I allow for a good balance of "doing" energy and "being" energies?
- What can I do to help my future self out?
- What works?
- What doesn't work?
- What is something I can do differently the next time to get a more positive result?
- Which archetype or archetypes would help me most in this situation?
- What sort of routines could be fun to implement to create more connection with myself and my family?
- What am I wanting or needing?
- What would my self care menu look like?
- What is perfect about this?
- What is this trying to teach me or help me practice?
- What brings me joy?
- What makes me happy to see?
- What are my favorite scents?
- What do I love to eat?
- What are some things I love to feel?
- What do I enjoy listening to?
- Is there any way I can better this thing that I am avoiding or don't want to do?
- Is there something I am doing that I can take off of my plate either through a trade or payment?
- Are there things that I can let go of and not do?

PART SEVEN

A Hero's Journey in Parenting Conclusion

While this book is coming to an end, the Hero's Journey in Parenting continues.

Autism was what sent me on this hero's journey. I had crossed over the threshold of the known and though I didn't realize it at the time, it was going to teach me how to let go of the ideas I had about parenting and provide valuable lessons regarding what was best for our family.

This didn't come overnight and I actually tried incredibly hard to hold on to the way I thought things were going to go. It took some time to realize that things were going to be different for us, but once I allowed myself to grieve for the life I thought I was going to have, shift my perspective as a parent, and let go of expectations, the easier things became. This opened up so much possibility and was an incredibly freeing experience!

Acceptance allowed me to become more present in my life because I wasn't constantly scanning for other people's approval. I became more able to recognize all of the gifts our son brought to our lives that I hadn't noticed or fully appreciated. He is an amazing teacher for everyone who is blessed to be in his life.

You also have an amazing teacher in your life and it has been my intention to support you in navigating the life and the child that you have because, while it may not have been what you expected, it is reality. If you are open to it, you can learn some pretty powerful lessons on what actually matters in life.

Answering the call to adventure that is the essence of every hero's journey leads inevitably to becoming a new person, one who is more capable and empowered as a result of the challenges faced and lessons learned. I am beyond excited for you!!

I hope that you found what 1 shared helpful in your own hero's journey in parenting. It has been my intention to provide you with tools, questions and strategies that you have access to whenever they are needed. I have only shared what I actually use in my real, everyday life and I use these things constantly because my son is always growing and changing—and so am I!

You too can revisit these tools or strategies with new eyes, new perspectives and they can help you to get clarity around what is actually going on. From there, you can use your energy in effective and efficient ways in order to help yourself and your family.

We began with the realization that the threshold had been crossed into this unique Hero's Journey in Parenting. Noticing what you might have experienced as a result of this - battling reality with the hope of returning to a life that makes more sense and that feels easier to navigate - and how regardless of how much energy is spent doing so, it doesn't work. Accepting this and being open to a new approach, that has nothing to do with your child being any different, is where possibility for positive change and growth as a parent enters.

From there, seeds of awareness were planted about the Shadow Forces (the Storyteller, the Battle Ready Bodyguard and the Guardian of the Heart) and learning that while they are trying to be helpful, their "shadowy" ways just keep you stuck. Building a new relationship with them, using their talents and gifts in positive ways can allow them to support you so that you can support your child.

It is also important to recognize that there are Hindering Forces (mainly control and judgment) that are also trying to keep you safe but take precious time, energy and attention away from what actually matters. Becoming aware of when and how these Hindering Forces are activated can empower you to "see" them for what they are in order to make choices that are best for you and your child from a place of clarity and not out of fear.

We couldn't leapfrog over the Shadow and Hindering Forces because doing so would keep us from all of the goodness that the Empowering Forces bring! Utilizing them can help you to find greater ease and joy in your life so that you can feel more confident, content and happy. This shift in energy will be felt by all who are around you and while you cannot change reality, you can change how you approach it.

As I stated at the beginning of this book, it is my mission and passion to help people like you find a sense of ease, peace and joy while on this parenting journey because life is too short to feel isolated, judged, uncertain and exhausted.

You are NOT alone and I am honored to be on this Hero's Journey in Parenting with you.

Xoxo

Margaret

Acknowledgments

I have so much love and gratitude for my husband K. Michael who is always supportive of my passions and asked the questions I didn't want to hear that helped turn this book into something better than I could ever have imagined. That's how he does everything and I'm so glad he is my partner in life!

Thank you to people who have offered editing suggestions throughout the years - Houkje Ross, Jill Farmer, Katie Hanus, Clare Sanders, Marna Wohlfield, June Bayha. A special thanks to my father-in-law, William Webb, who helped bring this to the finish line.

Many thanks to the mentors, fellow coaches and friends who showed up for me with tools, questions and support along the way in my own hero's journey in parenting - June Bayha, Katie Hanus, Michael Trotta, Martha Beck, Jill Farmer, Debbie Reber, Sarah Bamford Seidelmann, Marna Wohlfield, Clare Sanders, Julie Puentes, Kelley Wolf, Eryn McEwan, Houkje Ross, Leslie Saunderlin, Alexis Pershall Robin, Indrani Goradia, Bridgette Parent, Stacy Vinciguerra, Angie Balmer, Nancy Baden, Nikki Nichols, Katie Griffin Gaston, Natalie Leonard, all of our KidVentures Therapists, Capitol School of Austin teachers, and many more. Without you, your wisdom, encouragement, and inspiration, I wouldn't have been able to weave everything together to create for others what I so badly needed when I began my own parenting journey.

For all of those who are part of my "Parenting the Child" and "Differently Wired" family, I love you so much! You have my heart always and I am here for you, cheering you on 100%. Thank you from the bottom of my heart for your trust and bravery in trying something new and a bit outside of the box when you chose to be part of this group. You have wonderful teachers in your lives, and they are so lucky to have you as their parents!!

Grateful for my family, some of whom are no longer with us on Earth, who have supported us in so many different ways throughout our journey. In abc order, because you know, family! Judy Ann Achey, Eileen Brown, Ellen and Patrick Donley, Tim and Andrea Donley, Mary Jones, Kerry Marsh, the "Paw Patrol" (aka Andrew's cousins Parker, Chase, Brayden and Easton), Chris and Jaymes Salestrom, Jody and Judy Vass, William and Angela Webb, Patty Wilkum, Amy and Gary Yost, Ginger and Tom Yost.

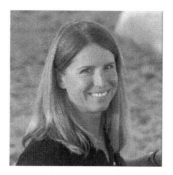

About the Author

Margaret Webb began her journey studying early childhood and elementary education at the University of Dayton. She went on to teach Kindergarten and Third Grade. After hitting rock bottom during her parenting journey, Margaret attended several life-changing retreats. Amazed at the impact of what she learned to support herself as a parent, she went on to become a Master Certified Martha Beck Life Coach, Sagefire Institute Nature Based Coach and Equus Trained Coach (uncertified).

This journey provided tools that changed her life as a person and parent and she created a course "Parenting the Child You Didn't Expect While You Were Expecting" that has helped hundreds of parents. In addition to her own coaching practice, she has been the parent coach for the "Differently Wired" club since its inception.

She currently resides in Austin, TX with her husband, son and three Jack Russell Terriers.

MargaretWebbLifeCoach.com

Made in the USA
Columbia, SC
12 March 2024

32505726R00248